Critical
Care
Notes

3rd Edition

Clinical Pocket Guide

Janice Jones, PhD, RN, CNS
Brenda Fix, DNP, RN, FNP-BC

Purchase additional copies of this book at your
health scie...
by shoppi...
calling 800...

D0713754

F.A. Davis Company • Philadelphia

F. A. Davis Company
1915 Arch Street
Philadelphia, PA 19103
www.fadavis.com

Printed in China

Last digit indicates print number: 10 9 8 7 6 5

Publisher, Nursing: Lisa B. Houck
Manager of Project and eProject Management: Catherine H. Carroll
Senior Content Project Manager: Christine M. Abshire
Illustration and Design Manager: Carolyn O'Brien

Reviewers: Katrina Allen-Thomas, MSN, CCRN, RN; Marilu Alltop, MSN, RN, CNE; Mallory Antico, MSN, RN; Lisa Ann Behrend, RN, MSNc, CCRN-CSC; Cynthia Berry, RN, DNP, CNE; Laura Carousel, MSN, RN, CCRN; Melanie Cates, RN, HBScN, MSN, ENC(C); Nancy L. Denny, MSN, RN-BC; Abimbola Farinde, PharmD, MS; Sarah Gabua, MSN, RN; Jayme Haynes, MSN, RN; Jeanie Krause-Bachand, MSN, EdD, RN, BC; Janice Garrison Lanham, RN, MSN, CCNS, FNP; Deborah Little, MSN, RN, CCRN, CNRN, APRN, BC; Angela Medina, RN, MSN; Candi Miller-Morris, MSN, RN, CNS, CCRN, CEN, TNS; Michelle Murphy-Rozanski, PhD, MSN, RN, CRNP; Deborah Pool, MS, RN, CCRN; Margaret Sherer, MS, RN, CEN, CNE; Denise A. Tucker, DSN, RN, CCRN; Tamra Weimer, RN, MS, CCRN, CNE; Danette Wood, EdD, MSN, RN, CCRN; Shawn Zembles, DNP, RN, CCRN, ACNS-BC

As new scientific information becomes available through basic and clinical research, recommended treatments and drug therapies undergo changes. The author(s) and publisher have done everything possible to make this book accurate, up to date, and in accord with accepted standards at the time of publication. The author(s), editors, and publisher are not responsible for errors or omissions or for consequences from application of the book, and make no warranty, expressed or implied, in regard to the contents of the book. Any practice described in this book should be applied by the reader in accordance with professional standards of care used in regard to the unique circumstances that may apply in each situation. The reader is advised always to check product information (package inserts) for changes and new information regarding dose and contraindications before administering any drug. Caution is especially urged when using new or infrequently ordered drugs.

Sticky Notes

✓HIPAA Compliant
✓OSHA Compliant

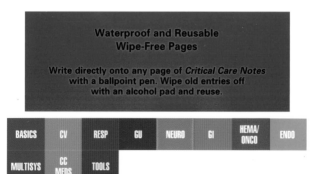

Waterproof and Reusable
Wipe-Free Pages

Write directly onto any page of *Critical Care Notes*
with a ballpoint pen. Wipe old entries off
with an alcohol pad and reuse.

BASICS	CV	RESP	GU	NEURO	GI	HEMA/ONCO	ENDO
MULTISYS	CC MEDS	TOOLS					

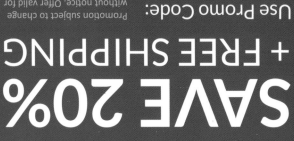

Physical Assessment

Reusable Assessment Form

Pt. Identifier:	Room:	Age:
Diagnosis:		
Surgeries/Past Hx:		
Activity:	Diet:	DNR/DNI:
Allergies:		
Neurological/MS: ICP:		
Cardiac: VS/A-line: ECG: Hemodynamics: PAD PAS PCWP CVP IABP:		
Respiratory: Ventilator: ABGs/SpO$_2$:		
GI:		
GU:		
Wounds/Incisions:		
Drainage tubes:		
Treatments:		
Special needs:		
Religion/Other:		

Normal Arterial and Venous Blood Gases

Blood Gas Components	Arterial	Venous
pH	7.35–7.45	7.31–7.41
PO_2	80–100 mm Hg	35–40 mm Hg
PCO_2	35–45 mm Hg	41–51 mm Hg
HCO_3^-	22–26 mEq/L or mmol/L	22–26 mEq/L or mmol/L
Base excess (BE)	–2 to +2 mEq/L or mmol/L	–2 to +2 mEq/L or mmol/L
O_2 saturation	95%–100%	68%–77%

Values denoted are at sea level.

Quick Blood Gas Interpretation

Acid-Base Disorder	pH	PCO_2	↑ HCO_3^-
Respiratory acidosis	↓	↑	↑ if compensating
Respiratory alkalosis	↑	↓	↓ if compensating
Metabolic acidosis	↓ and (+) base excess	↓ if compensating	↓
Metabolic alkalosis	↑ and (–) base excess	↑ if compensating	↑
Mixed respiratory and metabolic acidosis	↓	↑	↓
Mixed respiratory and metabolic alkalosis	↑	↓	↑

Full or total compensation: pH will be within normal limits.

Blood Gas Results

Arterial		Venous
	pH	
	Po_2	
	Pco_2	
	HCO_3^-	
	Base excess (BE)	
	O_2 saturation	

Compensation:

- Respiratory problem → the kidneys compensate by conserving or excreting HCO_3^-
- Metabolic problem → the lungs compensate by retaining or blowing off CO_2

Also look for mixed respiratory and metabolic problems. $Paco_2$ or HCO_3^- in a direction opposite its predicted direction or not close to predictive value. May result from cardiac arrest, vomiting with renal failure and COPD as comorbidities, and salicylate toxicity.

Common Causes of Acid-Base Imbalances

Respiratory acidosis	COPD, asthma, head injury, pulmonary edema, aspiration, pneumonia, ARDS, pneumothorax, cardiac arrest, respiratory depression, CNS depression, or head injury
Respiratory alkalosis	Hyperventilation, anxiety, fear, pain, fever, sepsis, brain tumor, mechanical overventilation
Metabolic acidosis	Diabetes mellitus, acute and chronic renal failure, severe diarrhea, alcoholism, starvation, salicylate overdose, pancreatic fistulas
Metabolic alkalosis	Loss of gastric acid (vomiting, gastric suction), long-term diuretic therapy (thiazides, furosemide), excessive $NaHCO_3$ administration, hypercalcemia

Pulse Oximetry

Spo₂ monitoring may be intermittent or continuous. Indirectly monitors oxygen saturation.

Spo₂ Level	Indication
<95%	Normal
91%–94%	May be acceptable, provide O₂ as necessary, encourage C&DB, or suction prn
85%–90%	Provide O₂ as necessary, encourage C&DB, or suction prn; may be normal for COPD patient
<85%	Prepare for possible intubation
<70%	Unreliable; obtain ABG

Values denoted are at sea level.

False readings may occur because of anemia, carbon monoxide poisoning, hypothermia, hypovolemia, hypotension, peripheral vasoconstriction, and poor peripheral perfusion caused by disease or medications.

Continuous Monitoring

- Alarms are set for low Spo₂, tachycardia, or bradycardia.
- Waveform should be sharp with a clearly identified dicrotic notch.
- The probe may be placed on the finger (preferred), toes, or ear lobe or pinna.
- Patient must have SBP >80 mm Hg.

Lactic Acidosis

Lactic acid is a byproduct of anaerobic metabolism. Increased levels indicate inadequate perfusion of vital organs with resultant tissue hypoxia. May result from inadequate perfusion and oxygenation of vital organs; post cardiac or respiratory arrest; cardiogenic, ischemic, or septic shock; drug overdoses; seizures; cancers; or diabetes mellitus (refer to Multisystem tab).

Normal lactate level <2 mmol/L; >5 mmol/L indicates lactic acidosis.

Respiratory Terms and Calculations

- Functional residual capacity (FRC) is the volume of air in the lungs after normal expiration.
  Normal = 2,400 mL.
- Hypoxemia is the severe reduction of O_2 in arterial blood.
- Hypoxia is the severe reduction of O_2 at the cellular level.
- Minute ventilation (MV) = respiratory rate (RR) × tidal volume (V_T).
  To improve MV and ↓ $PaCO_2$ with mechanical ventilation: ↑ V_T, and/or ↑ RR; ↑ inspiratory pressure, prolong inspiratory time, ↑ pressure support level, ↓ airway resistance, suctioning, use of bronchodilators.
- P/F (PaO_2/FIO_2) ratio. The smaller the value, the worse the patient's gas exchange. Frequently calculated to suggest ARDS and V̇/Q̇ mismatch.
  Normal = 300–500; impending or actual respiratory failure = 200–300 (may need to intubate); ARDS or V̇/Q̇ mismatch = <200, indicates hypoxemia and need to intubate.
  Formula: PaO_2 (from ABG in mm Hg) ÷ FIO_2 (converted to decimal) = P/F ratio number.
  Example: PaO_2 = 87 mm Hg and patient is on room air (21% = 0.21) = 77 ÷ 0.21 = 366.
- SaO_2 is the saturation of oxygen in hemoglobin in arterial blood = 95%–100% normal. Obtained from arterial blood sample.
- SvO_2 is the percentage of O_2 bound to hemoglobin in venous blood = 60%–80%. Assesses tissue perfusion or oxygenation of tissues. May be monitored intermittently or continuously using an oximetric pulmonary artery catheter. $ScvO_2$ is a central venous sample from internal jugular or subclavian catheters = >70%.
  ↑ SvO_2 (>80%) indicates an ↑ in O_2 delivery or ↓ O_2 extraction by tissues.
  ↓ SvO_2 (<60%) indicates a ↓ in O_2 delivery or ↑ extraction by tissues
  → cardiac output not adequate to meet tissue O_2 needs; Hgb may be low; O_2 consumption > oxygen delivery.

End-Tidal Carbon Dioxide Monitoring (ETco₂)

$ETCO_2$ or capnography/capnometry is the measurement, display, and monitoring of the concentration or partial pressure of CO_2 ($ETCO_2$) in the respiratory gases at the end of expiration. $ETCO_2$ values are usually 2–5 mm Hg lower than the $PaCO_2$ value. The capnogram displays the maximum inspiratory and expiratory CO_2 concentrations during a respiratory cycle that indirectly reflect the production of CO_2 by the tissues and the transport and clearance of CO_2 to and in the lungs. Sudden changes in CO_2 elimination should be monitored in selected cardiorespiratory patients and postoperatively after major cardiothoracic surgery.

ETCO$_2$ monitoring can also be used to verify ETT position, assess readiness for extubation, and monitor the effectiveness of CPR and predict patient survival. ETCO$_2$ <10 mm Hg after 20 min CPR indicates poor outcome. It is sometimes referred to as the "ventilation vital sign."

Causes of ↓ ETCO$_2$	Causes of ↑ ETCO$_2$
Fever	Hypothermia
Hypertension	Hypotension and shock
Increased cardiac output	Cardiac perfusion changes
Hypoventilation	Decreased cardiac output, heart failure
Respiratory compromise	Cardiac arrest and apnea
Hyperventilation	Airway obstruction
Airway obstruction	Hyperventilation
Bronchial intubation	Accidental extubation
Hypovolemia	Pulmonary embolus
Sepsis	Sepsis
Seizures	Hypervolemia

Normal range of ETCO$_2$ is 35–45 mm Hg. CO$_2$ and ETCO$_2$ should correlate with-in 2–5 mm Hg.

↑ RR (hyperventilation) → ↑ CO$_2$ → ETCO$_2$ < 35 = respiratory alkalosis
↑ RR (hypoventilation) → ↓ CO$_2$ → ETCO$_2$ > 45 = respiratory acidosis

Five characteristics of the capnogram should be evaluated: frequency, rhythm, height, and shape. Also note changes if patient is disconnected from ventilator and attempts of spontaneous breaths if patient is receiving paralytic agents.

Normal Capnogram

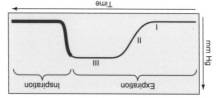

Phases I, II, and III represent expiration; the bolded lines represent inspiration. Long periods of a flat waveform indicate apnea, dislodged endotracheal tube, esophageal intubation, or patient disconnection from ventilator.

Artificial Airways and Mechanical Ventilation

Artificial Airways

Endotracheal Tube
- Adult oral tube sizes: males, 8.0–8.5 internal diameter (I.D.) (mm); females, 7.0–8.0. I.D. (mm).
- Placement is 2–3 cm above the carina. Verify by auscultating for breath sounds bilaterally, uniform up-and-down chest movement, CXR, and checking $ETCO_2$ immediately after intubation.
- Cuff pressure: 20–25 mm Hg.

  Rapid Sequence Induction (RSI): Minimizes time to intubation and secures a patent airway. Beforehand, differentiate if a surgical airway is needed instead.

- Procedure outline:
  - Preoxygenate patient with 100% O_2.
  - Induction drug administered: etomidate, propofol, ketamine, thiopental, or scopolamine.
  - Neuromuscular blocking agent administered: succinylcholine or rocuronium.
  - Apply cricoid pressure (Sellick maneuver) to minimize gastric aspiration.
  - ETT inserted.
- Nursing concerns:
  - Know patient's K^+ level.
  - Have routine intubation supplies available.
  - Check for workable suction source and provide regular suction catheter and Yankauer catheter.
  - Provide emotional support to patient and notify patient's family of rapid induction of ETT.

  Cuff pressure can be monitored via a calibrated aneroid manometer device. Connect manometer to cuff. Deflate cuff. Reinflate cuff in 0.5-mL increments until desired cuff pressure is achieved. Check cuff pressure every 8–12 hr or per agency protocol.

Tracheostomy Tube
- Tracheostomy tubes may be cuffed or uncuffed and have either a reusable or disposable inner cannula. Both fenestrated and Passy-Muir valves allow the patient to speak.
- Size will vary.
- Cuff pressure: 20–25 mm Hg.
- Early replacement of ETT with tracheotomy has not been shown to improve patient outcomes.
- Other artificial airways include oropharyngeal airway and nasopharyngeal airway.

Oxygen delivery systems include the nasal cannula, face mask, Venturi mask, partial rebreather mask, nonrebreather mask, tracheostomy collar, and T-piece.

- Nonrebreather mask allows for 80%–90% FiO_2 to treat lowing O_2 levels as exhibited by decreasing SpO_2 or impending respiratory failure prior to intubation.
- The T-piece may be connected to either an ETT or a tracheostomy tube. Frequently used in ventilator weaning.

Mechanical Ventilation

Classification of Ventilators
Positive Pressure Ventilation
- **Volume-Cycled Ventilator:** Delivers a preset constant volume of air and preset O_2.
- **Pressure-Cycled Ventilator:** Produces a flow of gas that inflates the lung until the preset airway pressure is reached.
- **Time-Cycled Ventilator:** Programmed to deliver a volume of gas over a specific time period through adjustments in inspiratory-to-expiratory ratio. Primarily used in neonates.

Negative Pressure Ventilation
Uses the old iron lung principle by exerting negative pressure on the chest wall to cause inspiration. No intubation required. Custom-fitted "cuirass" or "turtle" shell unit fits over the chest wall. May be used at night for patients who require assistance during sleep.

Modes of Ventilation
- **Continuous Mandatory Ventilation (CMV):** Machine controls rate of breathing. Delivery of preset volume (TV) and rate regardless of patient's breathing pattern. Sedation or neuromuscular blocking agent usually required. Very restricted use (e.g., SCI).
- **Assist Controlled Ventilation (AC or ACV):** Patient controls rate of breathing. Inspiratory effort triggers delivery of preset volume.
- **Synchronized Intermittent Mandatory Ventilation (SIMV):** A form of pressure support ventilation. Administers mandatory ventilator breath at a preset level of positive airway pressure. Monitors negative inspiratory effort and augments patient's spontaneous tidal volume or inspiratory effort. Synchronized with patient's breathing pattern.
- **Positive End-Expiratory Pressure (PEEP):** Increases oxygenation by increasing functional residual capacity (FRC). Keeps alveoli inflated after expiration. Can use lower O_2 concentrations with PEEP; decreases risk of O_2 toxicity. Ordered as 5–10 cm H_2O.
- **Pressure Support Ventilation (PS or PSV):** Patient's inspiratory effort is assisted by the ventilator to a certain level of pressure. Patient initiates

all breaths and controls flow rate and tidal volume. Decreases work of breathing and promotes weaning.
- **Pressure-Controlled Ventilation (PCV):** Controls plateau pressures in patients with ARDS and persistent oxygenation problems despite high levels of PEEP and FIO_2.
- **Pressure-Regulated Volume Control (PRVC):** Preset rate, FIO_2, and pressure limit. Improves patient-ventilator synchrony and reduces barotrauma. May require sedation.
- **Volume-Assured Pressure Support (VAPS) or Volume Guaranteed Pressure Options (VGPO):** Combination of pressure with guaranteed volume control.
- **High-Frequency Ventilation (HFV):** Delivers very high breaths/min with low tidal volumes. These include high-frequency oscillatory ventilation (**HFOV or HFO**), high-frequency jet ventilation (**HFJV**), and high-frequency positive pressure ventilation (**HFPPV**).
- **Inverse Ratio Ventilation (IRV):** All breaths are pressure limited and time cycled. Inspiratory time usually set shorter than expiratory time. I:E ratio is usually 1:1.3–1.5

Noninvasive Mechanical Ventilation (NIV)
- **Continuous Positive Airway Pressure (CPAP):** A form of noninvasive mechanical ventilation (NIMC). Maintains positive pressure throughout the respiratory cycle of a spontaneously breathing patient. Increases the amount of air remaining in the lungs at the end of expiration. Fewer complications than PEEP. Ordered as 5–10 cm H_2O.
- **Bilevel Positive Airway Pressure (BiPAP):** Same as CPAP but settings can be adjusted for both inspiration and expiration.

SIMV, CPAP, BiPAP, and PSV can all be used in the weaning process.

General Nursing Care for Mechanically Ventilated Patients
- General routine head-to-toe assessment to monitor for complications related to mechanical ventilation.
- Check ventilator settings for accuracy, especially rate, tidal volume, FIO_2, PEEP level, and pressure gauge; monitor ABGs after ventilator setting changes.
- Assess for oxygen toxicity. Cellular damage causing capillary leak → pulmonary edema and ARDS. May develop if patient on 100% FIO_2 for >12 hr or >50% FIO_2 for >24 hr. Monitor for dyspnea, ↑ lung compliance, ↓ A-a gradient, paresthesia in the extremities, and retrosternal pain. Keep O_2 at lowest possible concentration. Consider PEEP to ↑ FIO_2. If patient is anemic, transfuse RBCs.
- Administer analgesics, sedation drugs, and neuromuscular blocking agents as needed.

- Provide communication methods for patients, and communicate freely with families.
- Prevent infection including catheter-associated urinary tract infection (CAUTI), central catheter-associated bloodstream infection (CLABSI), and ventilator-associated pneumonia (VAP) (refer to VAP guidelines in Respiratory tab).
- Assess readiness to wean.

Weaning
Sample Criteria for Weaning: Readiness
- Alert and cooperative
- FIO_2 <40%–50% and PEEP <5–8 cm H_2O
- Hemodynamically stable with HR <120 bpm and no significant arrhythmias, SBP >100 mm Hg
- pH >7.34
- PaO_2 >80 mm Hg
- $PaCO_2$ <45 mm Hg
- PaO_2/FIO_2 ratio >200
- $ETCO_2$ <40 mm Hg
- Vital capacity 15 mL/kg and minute ventilation <10
- Hemoglobin >7–9 g/dL and serum electrolytes within normal limits
- Spontaneous respirations >6 bpm or <35 bpm
- Negative inspiratory pressure –30 cm H_2O
- Relatively afebrile with limited respiratory secretions and good cough reflex
- Good pain management
- Inotropes reduced or unchanged within previous 24 hr
- Sedation discontinued
- Spontaneous breathing trials (SBT)

Weaning Protocol	
Hospital Weaning Protocol	**Patient's Readiness for Weaning**

Continued

Weaning Protocol—cont'd	
Hospital Weaning Protocol	**Patient's Readiness for Weaning**

Weaning Methods

- **T-tube weaning:** Place patient on T-tube circuit on same FiO_2 as on ventilatory assistance. Monitor ABGs after 30 min. Provide a brief rest period on the ventilator as needed and continue to monitor ABGs until satisfactory. Extubate when patient is rested, has good spontaneous respiratory effort, and ABGs within acceptable parameters.
- **SIMV weaning:** Decrease SIMV rate every 1–4 hr or 2 breaths/min. Monitor spontaneous breaths, SpO_2 with a goal of >90%, $ETCO_2$, hemodynamics, and ECG for dysrhythmias. Obtain ABGs within 30 min of ventilator change. Allows for gradual change from positive pressure ventilation to spontaneous pressure ventilation. Titrate FiO_2.
- **PSV:** Use low levels of PSV (5–10 cm H_2O). Decrease in 3–6 cm of H_2O increments. Useful in retraining respiratory muscles from long-term ventilation.
- **CPAP/BiPAP:** Provides expiratory support, maintains positive intrathoracic pressure. BiPAP adds inspiratory support to CPAP. Prevents respiratory muscle fatigue.

Nursing Assessment During Weaning

- Vital signs and hemodynamic stability (PAS, PAD, PCWP, CO, CI)
- Dysrhythmias or ECG changes
- Oxygenation/efficiency of gas exchange: SaO_2 >90% on <40% FiO_2
- CO_2 production and elimination
- pH level
- Bedside pulmonary function tests
- Work of breathing including use of accessory muscles
- Adequate clearing of airway though effective coughing
- Level of fatigue
- Patient discomfort
- Adequate nutrition

Ventilator Alarms

Ventilator alarms should never be ignored or turned off. They may be muted or silenced temporarily until problem is resolved.

Checklist of Common Causes of Ventilator Alarms

Patient causes:

- Biting down on endotracheal tube
- Patient needing suctioning
- Coughing
- Gagging on endotracheal tube
- Patient "bucking," or not synchronous with the ventilator
- Patient attempting to talk
- Patient experiencing period of apnea >20 sec
- Development of pneumothorax from increasing intrathoracic pressures

Mechanical causes:

- Kinking of ventilator tubing
- Endotracheal tube cuff may need more air
- Leak in endotracheal tube cuff
- Excess water in ventilator tubing
- Leak or disconnect in the system
- Air leak from chest tube if present
- Malfunctioning of oxygen system
- Loss of power to ventilator

Pathophysiological causes:

- Increased lung noncompliance, such as in ARDS
- Increased airway resistance, such as in bronchospasm
- Pulmonary edema
- Pneumothorax or hemothorax

Nursing Interventions

- Check ventilator disconnects and tubing.
- Assess breath sounds; suction as needed.
- Remove excess water from ventilator tubing.
- Check endotracheal cuff pressure.
- Insert bite block or oral airway.
- If cause of the alarm cannot be found immediately or cause cannot be readily resolved, remove patient from ventilator and manually ventilate patient using a resuscitation (Ambu) bag.
- Call respiratory therapy stat.
- Continue to assess patient's respiratory status until mechanical ventilation is resumed.

Implementing the ABCDEF Bundle at the Bedside From the American Association of Critical Care Nurses

The ABCDEF bundle is a group of evidence-based practices that help prevent unintended consequences in critically ill patients. Detailed guidelines can be found at: www.icudelirium.org/medicalprofessionals.html

The ABCDEF bundle consists of:

A—Assess, Prevent, and Manage Pain using the Behavioral Pain Scale & the Critical-Care Pain Observation Tool

B—Both Spontaneous Awakening Trials and Spontaneous Breathing Trials should be attempted with assistance from respiratory therapist. Use "sedation vacations" to promote earlier extubation as coordinated with pharmacist.

C—Choice of Analgesia and Sedation using the Richard Agitation-Scale & the Analgesia/Sedation Protocol for Mechanically Ventilated Patients

D—Delirium Assessment, Prevention, and Management: Early identification and management of patients with delirium using the CAM-ICU or the Intensive care Delirium Screening Checklist.

E—Early Exercise and Progressive Mobility: Enable patients to become progressively more active and, possibly, walk while intubated. Seek assistance from physical therapists.

F—Family Engagement and Empowerment. Allow liberal visiting hours and keep family well informed and involved in key decisions. Communicate frequently.

Analgesia/Sedation Protocol for Mechanically Ventilated Patients can be found at: http://www.icudelirium.org/docs/Sedation_protocol.pdf

Analgesics
Sedatives
Anxiolytics

Sedation weaning also includes:

- Use of short-term sedatives
- Daily sedation interruptions using the "Wake Up and Breathe" protocol. Refer to: http://www.icudelirium.org/docs/WakeUpAndBreathe.pdf
- Treatment of pain
- Use of sedation scales (refer to Basics tab on Sedation)
- Regular assessment of delirium using the CAM-ICU (refer to Basics tab on Delirium)

Ventilator Complications

Complication	Signs & Symptoms/Interventions
Barotrauma or volutrauma: acute lung injury, may result in pneumothorax or tension pneumothorax, pneumomediastinum, pneumoperitoneum, subcutaneous crepitus	High peak inspiratory and mean airway pressures Diminished breath sounds Tracheal shift Subcutaneous crepitus Hypoxemia Insert chest tube or needle thoracostomy.
Intubation of right mainstem bronchus	Absent or diminished breath sounds in left lung Unilateral chest excursion Reposition ETT.
Endotracheal tube out of position or unplanned extubation	Absent or diminished breath sounds Note location of tube at the lip (21–22 cm). Reposition ETT or reintubate. Restrain only when necessary.
Tracheal damage from excessive cuff pressure (>30 cm H_2O)	Blood in sputum when suctioning Frequent ventilator alarm Monitor ETT cuff pressure every 4–8 hr. Ensure minimal occluding volume.
Damage to oral or nasal mucosa	Skin breakdown or necrosis to lips, nares, or oral mucous membranes Reposition tube side-side of mouth every day. Apply petroleum jelly to nares. Provide oral care with toothbrush every 2 hr. Follow VAP protocol for oral care.
Aspiration Tracheoesophageal fistulas	Feeding viewed when suctioning Keep head of bed 30–45 degrees. Administer proton pump inhibitors or histamine H_2-receptor antagonists. Blue dye in feeding not recommended.
Ventilator-associated pneumonia Respiratory infection Increased risk of sinusitis	Refer to Respiratory section on VAP Assess color and odor of sputum. Monitor temperature, WBC count, ESR.

Continued

Ventilator Complications—cont'd

Complication	Signs & Symptoms/Interventions
Decreased venous return → decreased cardiac output from increased intrathoracic pressure	Hypotension Decreased CVP, RAP, and preload Monitor vital signs and hemodynamics.
Stress ulcer and GI bleeding Gastric distention	Blood in nasogastric drainage Hematemesis and/or melena Hematest nasogastric drainage, emesis, feces. Administer proton pump inhibitors or histamine H_2-receptor antagonists. Auscultate bowel sounds. Consider NG placement.
Paralytic ileus	Absence of diminished bowel sounds Provide nasogastric drainage with intermittent suction. Turn and position patient frequently.
Inadequate nutrition, loss of protein	Refer to section on nutrition. Start enteral feedings if appropriate. Start total parenteral nutrition if GI tract nonfunctional or contraindicated.
Increased intracranial pressure	Changes in level of consciousness Inability to follow commands Assess neurological status frequently.
Fluid retention from increased humidification from ventilator, increased pressure to baroreceptors causing release of ADH	Assess for edema. Administer diuretics. Drain ventilator tubing frequently.
Immobility Skin breakdown	Turn and position patient frequently. Assess skin for breakdown. Assist patient out of bed to chair unless contraindicated. Keep skin clean and dry, sheets wrinkle-free.

Continued

Ventilator Complications—cont'd

Complication	Signs & Symptoms/Interventions
Communication difficulties	Keep communication simple. Obtain slate or writing board. Use letter/picture chart. Communicate using sign language.
Urinary tract infection	Urine becoming cloudy, concentrated, odorous Change/remove Foley catheter. Ensure adequate hydration. Administer anti-infectives.
Deep vein thrombosis	Painful, swollen leg; pain may increase on dorsiflexion Assess for pulmonary embolism. Refer to Respiratory tab. Administer heparin or enoxaparin.
Psychosocial concerns: fear, loss, powerlessness, pain, anxiety, sleep disturbances, nightmares, loneliness	Anxiety Difficulty sleeping Poor pain control Administer anxiolytics, sedatives, analgesics. Cluster activities to promote periods of sleep. Allow patient to make choices when appropriate. Allow for frequent family visits. Keep patient and family informed.

Neuromuscular Blocking Agents (NMBA)

Purposes
- Facilitate rapid sequence intubation.
- Facilitate mechanical ventilation and improve gas exchange.
- Reduce ICP.
- Control excessive shivering.
- Infusions may be used in intra-abdominal hypertension, complex head trauma, and ARDS as a last resort treatment.

Neuromuscular Blocking Agents and Induction Medications Used

- Atracurium (Tracium)
- Cisatracurium (Nimbex)
- Mivacurium
- Succinylcholine (Quelicin)
- Rocuronium (Zemuron)
- Pancuronium (Pavulon)
- Vecuronium

Peripheral Nerve Stimulator

- Monitors the level of blockade with NMBA use.
- Electrical stimulation is applied to the ulnar nerve (preferred), the facial nerve, or the posterior tibial nerve.
- Train of four (TOF) testing and monitoring should be instituted. The number of twitches elicited through electrodes along a nerve path is counted. Depth of blockage increases, number of twitches on the TOF decreases. Prevents overparalyzing the patient and causing prolonged muscular weakness.

Specific Nursing Management

- Patient **must** be intubated or have tracheostomy in place. Keep airway patent, and respond to ventilator alarms quickly.
- Monitor and assess response to NMBAs.
- Monitor VS and neurological status, especially pupillary response.
- Monitor ABGs and oxygenation levels.
- Provide eye lubrication and/or taping.
- Provide DVT prophylaxis.
- Initiate pressure sore prevention actions.

Hemodynamic Monitoring

Hemodynamic Parameters

Arteriovenous oxygen difference....................................3.5–5.5 vol% or 4–8 L/min
Aortic pressure:

- Systolic ....100–140 mm Hg
- Diastolic ....60–80 mm Hg
- Mean ....70–90 mm Hg

Cardiac output (CO = HR × SV)..4–8 L/min
Cardiac index (CO/BSA) ....2.5–4 L/min
Central venous pressure (CVP) ....2–8 mm Hg
**Same as right atrial pressure (RAP)
Cerebral perfusion pressure (CPP)..70–90 mm Hg

Coronary artery perfusion pressure (CAPP) ....60–80 mm Hg
Ejection fraction (Ej Fx or EF) 60%–75%
Left atrial mean pressure ....4–12 mm Hg
Left ventricular systolic pressure ....100–140 mm Hg
Left ventricular diastolic pressure ....0–5 mm Hg
Left ventricular end-diastolic pressure (LVEDP) ....5–10 mm Hg
Left ventricular end-diastolic volume (LVEDV) .... 120–130 mL up to 250 mL
Left ventricular stroke work index (LSWI) ....30–50 g/beats/m²
Mean arterial pressure (MAP) ....70–100 mm Hg
Mean arterial pressure used to determine whether BP is sufficient to perfuse
    the heart, brain, kidneys, and other organs
Oxygen consumption (VO₂) ....200–250 mL/min
Oxygen delivery (Do₂) ....900–1100 mL/min
Pulmonary artery pressure (PAP):

- Systolic ....20–30 mm Hg
- Diastolic ....10–20 mm Hg
- Mean ....10–15 mm Hg

Pulmonary capillary wedge pressure (PCWP) ....4–12 mm Hg
Pulmonary vascular resistance (PVR) ....37–250 dyne/sec/cm
Pulse pressure (SBP–DBP) ....40 mm Hg
Right atrial mean pressure ....2–6 mm Hg
Right ventricular pressure:

- Systolic ....20–30 mm Hg
- Diastolic ....0–8 mm Hg
- End diastolic ....2–6 mm Hg

Right ventricular stroke work index (RSWI) ....7–12 g/m²/beat
Pulmonary vascular resistance (PVR) .... 20–130 dynes/sec/cm⁻⁵
Pulmonary vascular resistance index (PVRI) ....200–400 dynes/sec/cm⁵/m²
Pulmonary ventricular stroke index ....5–10 g/beat/m²
Right atrial pressure (RAP) ....2–6 mm Hg
Stroke index (SI) ....30–650 mL/beat/m²
Stroke volume (SV = CO/HR) ....60–100 mL/beat
Systemic vascular resistance (SVR) ....900–1,600 dynes/sec/cm⁻⁵
Systemic vascular resistance index ....1,360–2,200 dynes/sec/cm⁻⁵/m²
Systemic venous oxygen saturation (SvO₂) 60%–80%

Cardiac Output Components

Preload	Contractility	Afterload
Pao_2	Sao_2	Hemoglobin (Hgb)
Right atrial pressure	Stroke volume	Pulmonary vascular resistance
Central venous pressure	Cardiac output	Systemic vascular resistance
Left ventricular end-diastolic pressure	Tissue perfusion	Blood pressure

Pulmonary Artery Catheter

The purpose of the pulmonary artery catheter, also known as the Swan-Ganz catheter, is to assess and monitor left ventricular function and can determine preload, assess contractility, and approximate afterload.

PCWP approximates left atrial pressure and left ventricular end-diastolic pressure.

Increases in PCWP, LAP, or LVEDP indicate heart failure, hypervolemia, shock, mitral valve insufficiency, or stenosis. Decreases in PCWP, LAP, or LVEDP indicate hypovolemia.

PA Catheter Waveforms

The pulmonary artery catheter is threaded through the right atrium and right ventricle and into the pulmonary artery. Insertion is done via fluoroscopy or monitoring waveform changes.

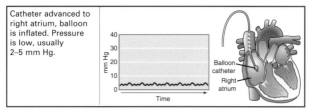

Catheter advanced to right atrium, balloon is inflated. Pressure is low, usually 2–5 mm Hg.

Continued

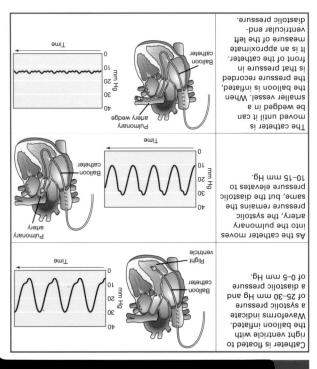

Catheter is floated to right ventricle with the balloon inflated. Waveforms indicate a systolic pressure of 25–30 mm Hg and a diastolic pressure of 0–5 mm Hg.

As the catheter moves into the pulmonary artery, the systolic pressure remains the same, but the diastolic pressure elevates to 10–15 mm Hg.

The catheter is moved until it can be wedged in a smaller vessel. When the balloon is inflated, the pressure recorded is that pressure in front of the catheter. It is an approximate measure of the left ventricular end-diastolic pressure.

Problems With Pulmonary Artery Catheters

Problem	Check For/Action
No waveform	• Loose connections • Tubing kinked or compressed • Air in transducer • Loose/cracked transducer • Stopcock mispositioned • Occlusion by clot: Aspirate as per policy
Overdamping (smaller waveform with slow rise, diminished or absent dicrotic notch)	• Air bubble or clot in the system • Catheter position: Reposition patient or have patient cough • Kinks or knotting • Clot: Aspirate as per policy
Catheter whip (erratic waveform, variable and inaccurate pressure)	• Catheter position: Reposition patient or catheter; obtain chest x-ray
Inability to wedge catheter (no wedge waveform after inflating balloon)	• Balloon rupture: Turn patient on left side; check catheter position for retrograde slippage

Complications of Pulmonary Artery Catheters
- Risk for infection
- Altered skin integrity
- Air embolism
- Pulmonary thromboembolism
- Cardiac tamponade
- Dysrhythmias
- Altered cardiopulmonary tissue perfusion from thrombus formation; catheter in wedged position leading to pulmonary infarction
- Catheter displacement/dislodgment
- Loss of balloon integrity or balloon rupture
- Pneumothorax
- Hemothorax
- Frank hemorrhage
- Pulmonary artery extravasation
- Pulmonary artery rupture

Other methods of monitoring hemodynamics are esophageal Doppler hemodynamic monitoring system, impedance-based hemodynamic monitoring, and the arterial pressure–based cardiac monitoring system.

- Select hemodynamic effects.

- Positive pressure mechanical ventilation → increase in intrathoracic
  pressure and increase in right atrial pressure (RAP) → decrease in venous
  return (VR) → decrease CVP → decrease in preload → decrease in stroke
  volume and cardiac output. Other conditions affecting reduced preload
  include hemorrhage, hypovolemia.

Intra-Arterial Monitoring

An arterial line (A-line) is used if frequent blood pressure and arterial blood gas
determinations are needed. It is especially useful:

- After surgery.
- For patients with unstable vital signs.
- For patients experiencing hypoxemia.

Perform Allen's test prior to insertion. Elevate the patient's hand with his or
her fists clenched. Release pressure over only the ulnar artery. Color returns to
the hand within 6 sec if the ulnar artery is patent and adequate collateral blood
flow present.

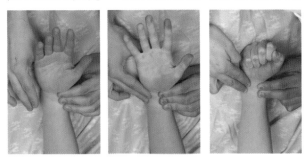

Compressing the radial and ulnar arteries

Observing for pallor

Releasing pressure and observing for return of normal color

Intra-Arterial Waveform

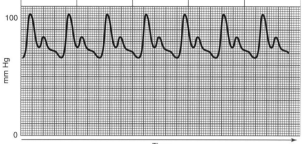

Components of Waveform

- **Systolic peak**: Ventricular ejection and stroke volume. Sharp rise and rounded top.
- **Dicrotic notch**: Aortic valve closure, end ventricular systole, start ventricular diastole. Should be one-third or greater of height of systolic peak. If lower → suspect ↓ CO.

Tapering of down stroke following dicrotic notch.

Important assessments: changes in capillary refill/blanching, sensation, motion, or color that may indicate lack of perfusion to the extremity.

$$MAP = \frac{systolic\ BP + (diastolic\ BP \times 2)}{3} = 70\text{–}100\ mm\ Hg$$

Decreased tissue perfusion—decreasing urine output, elevation in BUN:creatinine ratio, altered mental status with decreasing level of consciousness, restlessness, dyspnea, cyanosis, dysrhythmias, abnormal ABGs, weak or absent peripheral pulses, increased capillary refill time (>3 sec), diminished arterial pulsations, bruits.

Potential Complications of Intra-Arterial Monitoring

- Hemorrhage
- Air emboli
- Equipment malfunction/inaccurate pressure
- Dysrhythmias
- Infection
- Altered skin integrity
- Impaired circulation to extremities

Nutrition Issues in Critical Care

Primary Concerns

- Malnutrition, starvation, and catabolism
- Stress hypermetabolism
- Fluid volume deficit
- Fluid volume excess

Stress and Nutrition

Prolonged or continual stress depletes glycogen stores → hypermetabolic state.

Metabolic rate increases with the release of catecholamines + glucagon + cortisol → hyperglycemia and "stress diabetes."

Protein is lost via gluconeogenesis → decrease in serum protein (albumin).

Lipolysis → increase in free fatty acids.

Nitrogen excretion increases.

Body weight decreases.

1 kg body weight = 1 liter of fluid retained or lost.

Impaired immune function.

Body Mass Index

BMI is a simple means of classifying sedentary (physically inactive) individuals of average body composition and may indicate obesity. It is calculated by the following: Body mass index (BMI) = weight (kg) ÷ height (meters)^2

1 kg = 2.2 lb   Normal BMI = 20–25 kg/m^2

A BMI >30 kg/m^2 indicates obesity; >40 kg/m^2 indicates morbid obesity. An increase in BMI has been associated with heart disease and diabetes. A BMI <18.5 kg/m^2 suggests a person is underweight. A BMI <17.5 may indicate the person has anorexia or a related disorder.

BMI does not take into account factors such as frame size and muscularity.

Signs and Symptoms of Fluid Volume Deficit: Hypovolemia

- Dry mucous membranes; dry, coated, cracked, or fissured tongue
- Thirst; thick, scant saliva
- Poor skin turgor
- Sunken eyeballs
- Decreased or orthostatic blood pressure; narrow pulse pressure

- Weak, rapid heart rate and increased respiratory rate
- Decreased capillary refill
- Urine output decreased (<30 mL/hr)
- Increased specific gravity of urine (>1.030)
- Decreased central venous pressure
- Increased hemoglobin and hematocrit
- Increased BUN and serum osmolarity
- Increased BUN:creatinine ratio
- Lethargy, mental confusion

Signs and Symptoms of Fluid Volume Excess: Hypervolemia

- Crackles in lungs; dyspnea, shortness of breath → pulmonary congestion or pleural effusion
- Moist mucous membranes
- Full, bounding pulse; tachycardia
- Increased BP, CVP, and PAP
- Distended neck veins and jugular venous pressure
- Edema and decreased serum osmolarity; weight gain
- Decreased hemoglobin and hematocrit
- Decreased specific gravity of urine
- Mental confusion, restlessness

Management

- Intravenous fluids and volume expanders

Crystalloids
- Hypertonic: pulls fluid from the cell: $D_5/0.25\%$ NaCl, $D_5/0.45\%$ NaCl, $D_5/0.9\%$ NaCl, 3% NaCl, D_5/LR, D_{10}/W, $D_{50}W$
- Hypotonic: moves fluid into the cell: 0.45% NaCl, 2.5%D, D_5W
- Isotonic: improves hydration, post-op patients: D_5W, 0.9% NaCl, LR

Colloids
- Plasma or volume expanders: albumin (5% or 25%), or plasma protein, plasma protein fraction (Plasmanate) may have limited benefit

Enteral Tube Feedings

Early enteral nutrition has been shown to improve patient outcomes in critical care units and reduces ICU length of stay. Safe for patients after successful fluid resuscitation and correction of electrolyte imbalances. Separate IV infusions of the trace elements chromium, copper, manganese, selenium, and zinc have been shown to improve patient outcomes.

Types of Tube Feedings

- **Intermittent or bolus feedings:** A set volume of formula is delivered at specified times.
- **Continuous feedings:** A set rate of formula is delivered over a period of time.
- **Cyclic feedings:** Similar to a continuous feeding, but the infusion is stopped for a specified time within a 24-hr period, usually 6–10 hr.

Gastric Access
- Nasogastric tube (NGT)
- Oral
- Percutaneous endoscopic gastrostomy (PEG)
- Nasoduodenal tube (NDT)
- Low-profile gastrostomy device (LPGD)

Small Bowel Access
- Nasal-jejunal tube (NJT)
- Percutaneous endoscopic jejunostomy (PEJ)

The following are based on the Guidelines for the Provision and Assessment of Nutrition Support Therapy in the Adult Critically Ill Patient: Society of Critical Care Medicine (SCCM) and American Society for Parenteral and Enteral Nutrition (A.S.P.E.N.), 2016 Clinical Practice Guidelines:

- A nutritional screening score should be done within 48 hr of ICU admission (NUTRIC score).
- Nutrition support therapy should be instituted within the first 24–48 hr of ICU admission.
- In the ICU patient population, neither the presence nor absence of bowel sounds or evidence of passage of flatus and stool is required for the initiation of enteral feeding.
- In patients requiring significant hemodynamic support including high-dose catecholamine agents, alone or in combination with large-volume fluid or blood product resuscitation to maintain cellular perfusion, enteral nutrition should be withheld until the patient is fully resuscitated and/or stable.

Either small volume or full nutrition by enteral feeding is appropriate for patients with ARDS or acute lung injury and if the duration of mechanical ventilation is >/= 72 hr.

- Either gastric or small bowel feeding is acceptable in the ICU setting.

Nursing Care of the Patient Receiving Enteral Feeding
- Use hand hygiene and gloves when setting up or changing feeding administration set.
- Label with date, time, and nurse's name initials on all facets of the administration set.

- Sterile premixed formula should hang for <8 hr or per policy.
- Reconstituted formula exposed to room temperature should hang for <4 hr or per policy.
- Check expiration date on formula can.
- Change administration sets every 24 hr or per policy.
- Flush tube with water only; avoid juice and carbonated beverages.
- Flush tube with 30 mL water every 4 hr for continuous feedings, before and after intermittent feedings, and after checking residual volume measurement. Flush with 15–30 mL water before and after each medication administration.
- Keep HOB elevated 30°–45°.
- Consider hanging IV fluids at the head of the bed only. Use foot of the bed to hang enteral feedings.
- Assess and monitor serum glucose levels.
- Assess fluid and electrolyte status. Assess hydration.
- Reduce risk of aspiration or improve feeding tolerance by administering a prokinetic agent, use of chlorhexidine mouthwash, and elevating head of bed. Consider using lower GI tract for level of infusion.
- Vomiting, abdominal distention, high gastric residual, and diarrhea may be signs of GI intolerance to enteral nutrition.

Checking Tube Placement

Assessing tube placement continues to be controversial as caregivers try to balance reliability of accuracy and costs. The following are suggested methods for verifying enteral tube placement:

- Obtain chest x-ray or abdominal x-ray. Gold standard for verifying placement. **Always** obtain, and have someone verify, enteral tube placement after initial placement.
- Aspirate gastric contents and check pH.
  - Gastric aspirate pH 1–5 in fasting patients but may be as high as 6 if patient is taking medication to reduce gastric acid (famotidine, ranitidine, pantoprazole).
  - Commercially prepared formulas have a pH close to 6.6.
  - Respiratory secretions have pH >6.
  - Small intestine aspirate pH >6.
- Visually inspect gastric aspirate. May aspirate only feeding tube contents. Color varies.
- Mark location of exit site and note external tube length upon insertion of feeding tube. Does not necessarily indicate location of tube on subsequent inspections.
- Inject 20–30 mL of air into the tube while auscultating over the epigastrium below the diaphragm. Air in the stomach can be heard via a whooshing sound. Currently not recommended.

■ Two different placement checks are now recommended with each manipulation of the tube.

AACN Verification of Feeding Tube Placement Guidelines 2016: Use a variety (two or more) of bedside methods to check feeding tube location:

■ Observe for a change in length of the external portion of the feeding tube. Monitor tube position at 4-hr intervals.
■ Review routine CXR and abdominal x-ray reports.
■ Observe changes in volume and appearance of aspirate.
■ Measure pH of feeding tube aspirates.
■ Obtain an x-ray to confirm tube position when in doubt about tube's location.

Checking for Gastric Residual Volumes (GRVs)

1. Assess GRVs every 4 hr during initial 48 hr of feeding.
2. Gastric residual volumes should not be used routinely in monitoring ICU patients on enteral nutrition.
3. If GRVs still being measured, do not hold enteral feeds for residuals >500 mL unless other signs of intolerance are seen.
4. Administration of metoclopramide (Reglan) is not effective in reducing GRV.
5. Using a 30- to 60-mL syringe, withdraw gastric contents from the feeding tube. Note volume of formula. Flush with 30 mL water. Assess for pain, abdominal distention, "feeling full or bloated," nausea, and emesis. The following are based on the 2016 A.S.P.E.N. Enteral Nutrition Practice Recommendations.

Alternative strategies for GRV:

■ Daily physical exams to assess for tolerance.
■ Review of abdominal radiological films.
■ Daily evaluation of risk factors for aspiration.

Enteral Tube Feeding Complications

Mechanical Complications	Interventions
Nasopharyngeal discomfort	• Reposition tube.
Esophageal ulceration or bleeding esophageal varices	• Consider PEG or PEJ tube.
Clogged tube	• Flush with lukewarm water after every feeding. • Hospital protocol:

Continued

Enteral Tube Feeding Complications—cont'd

Mechanical Complications	Interventions
Tube displacement	• Reposition tube.
Extubation	• Insert new tube. • Consider PEG or PEJ tube.
Stomal leak or infection	• Keep area around stoma clean and dry.

Nonmechanical Complications	Interventions
Nausea, vomiting, cramps, bloating, abdominal distention	• Withhold or decrease amount, rate, and frequency of feedings. • Change to low-fat formula.
Diarrhea	• Withhold or decrease amount, rate, and frequency of feedings. • Change formula. • Administer psyllium fiber (Metamucil)
Aspiration	• Hold feedings. Check residuals. • Keep HOB elevated 30°–45° during feedings and 1 hr after bolus feedings
Gastric reflux	• Hold feedings. Check residuals. • Keep HOB elevated 30°–45°.
Dumping syndrome: nausea, vomiting, diarrhea, cramps, pallor, sweating, ↓ HR	• Withhold or decrease amount, rate, and frequency of feedings.

Total Parenteral Nutrition (TPN)

TPN is an IV solution of 10%–50% dextrose in water (CHO), amino acids (protein), electrolytes, and additives (vitamins, minerals, trace elements of insulin, vitamin K, zinc, famotidine). Fat emulsions provide fatty acids and calories. Solutions >10% dextrose must be infused via a central line.

- 1,000 mL 5% D/W contains 50 g sugar = <200 calories
- 1,000 mL 25% dextrose contains 250 g sugar = 1,000 calories

Indications

- Severe malnutrition
- Burns
- Bowel disorders (inflammatory disorders, total bowel obstruction, short bowel syndrome)
- Severe acute pancreatitis
- Acute renal failure
- Hepatic failure
- Metastatic cancer
- Postoperative major surgery if NPO >5 days

Nursing Care

- Each bag of TPN should be changed at least every 24 hr with tubing change.
- Monitor intake and output and weigh the patient daily.
- Monitor glucose levels, including finger stick blood sugars every 4 to 6 hr. Cover with regular insulin as necessary. If poor control of serum glucose, consider adding insulin to TPN and continue sliding scale coverage.
- Monitor serum electrolytes including magnesium, phosphate, triglycerides, prealbumin, transferrin, CBC, PT/PTT, and urine urea nitrogen.
- Assess IV site for redness, swelling, and drainage.
- Change gauze dressing around IV site every 48 to 72 hr, as per protocol. Transparent dressings may be changed every 7 days.
- If TPN is temporarily unavailable, hang 10% D/W at the same rate as TPN. Monitor for hypoglycemia.
- Place TPN on infusion pump. Monitor hourly rate. Never attempt to "catch up" if infusion not accurate.

Complications

Complications from TPN may be catheter related, mechanical, or metabolic.

Complications of TPN	Signs and Symptoms
Infection, catheter-related sepsis, septicemia, septic shock	Leukocytosis; fever; glucose intolerance; catheter site red, swollen, tender; drainage
Hypoglycemia blood glucose <70 mg/dL	Shaking, tachycardia, sweating, anxiety, dizziness, hunger, impaired vision, weakness, fatigue, headache, irritability
Hyperglycemia blood glucose >200 mg/dL	Extreme thirst, frequent urination, dry skin, hunger, blurred vision, drowsiness, nausea
Prerenal azotemia	$\uparrow$ BUN and serum Na$^+$, signs of dehydration, lethargy, coma

Continued

Nosocomial Infections in the ICU

Critical Care Risk Factors

- Nosocomial or hospital-acquired infections (HAIs) develop during hospitalization or up to 30 days post hospital discharge. They can prolong length of ICU stay; poor patient outcomes. Predisposing factors include:
  - Invasive lines and devices
  - Immunocompromising conditions
  - Serious underlying illness
  - Prolonged stay in critical care unit
  - Colonization and cross-infection
  - Mechanical ventilation
  - Overuse of antibiotics
  - Elderly status

Complications of TPN	Signs and Symptoms
Hepatic dysfunction	↑ serum liver function tests (SGOT, SGPT, alkaline phosphatase)
Pneumothorax, hydrothorax	SOB, restlessness, dyspnea, signs of hypoxia, chest pain
Subclavian/carotid artery puncture	radiating to back, arterial blood in syringe, tachycardia, pulsatile blood flow, bleeding from catheter site
Air embolus	Respiratory distress, dyspnea, SOB, tachycardia, ↓ BP, neurological deficits, cardiac arrest
Dysrhythmias	Atrial, junctional, and ventricular arrhythmias; ↑ C.O., ↓ BP, loss of consciousness
Hypo-/hypernatremia	Normal values: 135–145 mEq/L or 135–145 mmol/L
Hypo-/hyperkalemia	Normal values: 3.5–5.0 mEq/L or 3.5–5.0 mmol/L
Hypo-/hyperphosphatemia	Normal values: 3.0–4.5 mg/100 mL or 1.0–1.5 mmol/L
Hypo-/hypermagnesemia	Normal values: 1.5–2.0 mEq/L or 0.8–1.3 mmol/L
Hypo-/hypercalcemia	Normal values: 8.5–10.5 mg/100 mL or 2.1–2.6 mmol/L

Methicillin-Resistant *Staphylococcus Aureus* (MRSA)

Etiology
Transmitted by close contact with infected person. Health-care worker may be colonized with MRSA strain with absence of symptoms. The *Staphylococcus aureus* bacterium is resistant to methicillin, amoxicillin, penicillin, oxacillin, and other antibiotics.

Signs and Symptoms
- Skin infection: Boil or abscess, cellulitis
- Surgical wound: Swollen, red, painful, exudate (pus)
- Bloodstream: Fever, chills
- Lung infection/pneumonia: Shortness of breath, fever, chills
- Urinary tract: Cloudy urine, strong odor
- Infective carditis

Diagnosis
- Culture of infected area. Blood cultures may be necessary.

Treatment (Dosages vary depending on the source of infection & the patient's age and renal function.)
- Institute standard and contact precautions.
- Vancomycin (Vanocin, Vancoled) oral or IV; trough vancomycin levels the most accurate; monitoring of peak vancomycin levels not recommended
- Rifampin may be used in combination in select cases.
- Linezolid (Zyvox) 600 mg IV twice a day
- Daptomycin (Cubicin) 4 mg/kg/dose IV once daily
- Clindamycin 600 mg IV or orally three times a day

Clostridium Difficile (C-diff)

2016 Guidelines for Diagnosis, Treatment, and Prevention of *Clostridium difficile* Infections

Etiology
Clostridium difficile (C-diff) is a common cause of antibiotic-associated diarrhea (AAD) and is transmitted through the feces or any surface, device, or material that has become contaminated with feces.

Signs and Symptoms
- Watery diarrhea (at least 3 BMs/day for 2 or more days), rarely bloody. May be greenish, mucoid, and foul-smelling.
- Fever.
- Loss of appetite.

- Nausea.
- Crampy abdominal pain and lower abdominal tenderness.

Diagnosis

- Stool culture.
- CBC and serum chemistries.
- Glutamine dehydrogenase enzyme immunoassay (EIA).
- Abdominal x-rays, CT, and colonoscopy may also be indicated.

Treatment

- Discontinue current antibiotics. May give metronidazole (Flagyl) or oral or rectal (retention enema) or vancomycin to treat diarrhea depending on severity. Consider fidaxomicin (Dificid), which has also been shown to be more effective for cancer patients with C-diff instead of vancomycin and those resistant to vancomycin.
- Standard and contact precautions: Isolation in private room, gloves and gowns for personnel and visitors.
- Monitor fluid balance, electrolytes, albumin, and CBC.
- Alcohol-based rubs not effective. Soap-and-water hand hygiene recommended.
- Data do not support the use of probiotics or antiperistaltic agents. Bismuth subsalicylates may be helpful.
- Proton pump inhibitors (PPIs) may increase the incidence of C-diff–associated diarrhea.
- Opioids and loperamide may increase the risk of toxic megacolon.
- Opioids and loperamide may increase the risk of toxic megacolon.
- Consider fecal microbiota transplantation (FMT). Also referred to as fecal bacteriotherapy or fecal transplant. Hospital must have a procedure and protocol in place for implementation.
  - Healthy donor who meets select criteria.
  - Administer vancomycin preprocedure or per protocol.
  - Administer PPI the evening before and morning of procedure to reduce gastric acid or per protocol.
  - Donor stool is prepared into a fecal slurry.
  - Administered via colonoscopy, retention enema, or NG tube.
    - Average size adult: 50–200 mL via NG tube or 250–500 mL via colonoscopy.
  - To administer via NGT: Draw up slurry into 60-mL syringe and inject 50 mL/2–3 min.
    - Follow with 50 mL flush of NS.
  - Keep HOB elevated 30° or more for at least 2 hr post procedure.
  - Document diarrhea post procedure. Procedure may be repeated after 5 days.
- Consider adding cholestyramine (Questran) to drug regimen.
- Subtotal colectomy with preservation of the rectum may be indicated for severely ill patients with grossly elevated WBC and serum lactate levels.

Other Hospital-Acquired Infections of Concern in the ICU

- Catheter-associated urinary tract infections (CAUTI)
- Central line–associated bloodstream infections (CLABSI)
- Hospital-acquired pneumonia (non-VAP)
- Surgical site infections (SSI)
- Ventilator-associated pneumonia (VAP) (refer to Respiratory tab)

Psychosocial Issues in Critical Care

Environmental, Sensory Overload, and Sleep Deprivation

- **Sensory Overload:** A condition in which sensory stimuli are received at a rate and intensity beyond the level that the patient can accommodate.
- **Sensory Deprivation:** A condition in which the patient experiences a lack of variety and/or intensity of sensory stimuli.

Types of Sensory Stimuli
- Visual
- Auditory
- Kinesthetic
- Gustatory
- Tactile
- Olfactory

Signs and Symptoms of Sensory Problems
- Confusion
- Hallucinations
- Lethargy
- Behavioral changes (combativeness)
- Increased startle response
- Disorientation
- Anxiety
- Restlessness
- Panic
- Withdrawal
- Mood swings

Some of these same symptoms may be caused by select medications, especially in elderly patients. Refer to the Updated 2015 Beers Criteria for Potentially Inappropriate Medication Use in Older Adults from the American

Geriatrics Society at https://www.guideline.gov/summaries/49933/american-geriatrics-society-2015-updated-beers-criteria-for-potentially-inappropriate-medication-use-in-older-adults

- Other environmental and psychological concerns include noise, lights and color, sleep disturbances, lack of control, helplessness, hopelessness, spiritual distress, stress, anxiety, and fear.
- Nurses may suffer from alarm fatigue and moral distress.
- Psychiatric emergencies in the ICU include agitated delirium and psychosis, neuroleptic syndrome, serotonin syndrome, and psychiatric medication overdose.
- Palliative care protocols for the ICU are developing and include an interdisciplinary approach with the patient and family regarding withdrawal or withholding of advance care. Include family in rounds and scheduled meetings.
- A hospice model should be adopted, including symptom management to minimize discomfort, nutrition, hydration, dialysis, extubation, and spiritual care.
- Communication regarding the discontinuation of ICDs to prevent unwanted shocks.

Near-Death Experience

The experience of patients that they have glimpsed the afterlife when coming close to death. These perceptions may include:

- Seeing an intense light
- Seeing angels or departed loved ones
- Traveling through a tunnel

Out-of-Body Experience

The experience of being away from and overlooking one's body. The patient feels that the mind has separated from the body.

Family Needs of the Critical Care Patient

- Relief of anxiety
- Assurance of competent care
- Timely access to the patient
- Accurate and timely information about the patient's condition and prognosis in easily understandable terms
- Early notification of changes in the patient's condition
- Explanations regarding the environment, machinery, and monitoring equipment
- Honest answers to questions

- Emotional support
- Regard for the spiritual needs of the family and patient

Organ Donation

Transplantable organs include:

- Kidneys
- Heart
- Lungs
- Liver
- Pancreas
- Intestines

Corneas, the middle ear, skin, heart valves, bone, veins, cartilage, tendons, and ligaments can be stored in tissue banks and used to restore sight, cover burns, repair hearts, replace veins, and mend damaged connective tissue and cartilage in recipients.

Healthy adults between the ages of 18 and 60 yr can donate blood stem cells: marrow, peripheral blood stem cells, and cord blood stem cells.

Nursing Role in Organ Donation

- Provide accurate information regarding donation.
- Identify possible donors early.
- Work closely with the organ procurement organization and members of the health team to elicit donations.
- Provide emotional support to families considering donation, and make sure to respect their cultural and religious beliefs.
- Become a donor advocate among colleagues and for patients and their families.

General Criteria for Brain Death

- Absence of purposive movement
- Flaccid tone and absence of spontaneous or induced movements
- Persistent deep coma
- No response to pain
- Absence of spontaneous respiration
- Absence of brainstem reflexes:
- Midposition or pupils fixed and dilated
- No corneal, gag, or cough reflexes
- Absence of spontaneous oculocephalic (doll's eye phenomenon) reflex
- No vestibular response to caloric stimulation
- Isoelectric or flat electroencephalogram (EEG)
- Absent cerebral blood flow

These criteria vary from state to state.

Hemodynamic Management of Potential Brain-Dead Organ Donors

Ensure adequate intravascular volume and adequate cardiac output to ensure consistent perfusion to vital organs.

- ◼ MAP >60 mm Hg
- ◼ Urine output >1.0 mL/kg/hr
- ◼ Left ventricular ejection fraction >45%

Nursing Care

- ◼ Fluid management—fluids or diuretics
- ◼ Inotropic agents to correct low cardiac output
- ◼ Vasopressors to correct vasodilation
- ◼ Thyroid hormone
- ◼ Corticosteroids to reduce inflammation
- ◼ Vasopressin to support renal function
- ◼ Insulin to control glucose levels
- ◼ Regulate ventilator settings including use of PEEP
- ◼ Suction frequently to promote adequate oxygenation

Specific organ donation protocols:

_____

_____

_____

_____

_____

_____

_____

_____

_____

_____

_____

_____

Anxiety, Agitation, and Sedation

Purpose of sedation is to minimize use of neuromuscular paralysis agents. Short-term use will ↓ ventilatory time, ↓ length of stay in ICU, ↓ costs, lead to fewer tracheostomies, and provide early intervention of neurological deterioration.

Long-term use has the opposite effects. Contributing factors: stress, ICU environment, pain, sleep deprivation, surgery, and anesthesia. Anxiety and agitation can lead to delirium and changes in LOC with poorer patient outcomes.

Sedatives should be titrated without impairing neurological assessment.

Analgesics should be titrated to keep pain level <3 on 0–10 scale.

Assessment

Prior to sedation, exclude and treat possible causes of agitation and confusion:

- Cerebral hypoperfusion
- Cardiac ischemia
- Hypotension
- Hypoxemia or hypercarbia (elevated blood CO_2)
- Fluid and electrolyte imbalance: acidosis, hyponatremia, hypoglycemia, hypercalcemia, hepatic or renal insufficiency
- Infection
- Drug-induced agitation or confusion, especially in elderly patients
- Furosemide (Lasix) (can contribute to agitation)

Use nonpharmacological therapies such as repositioning, massage, distraction, minimizing of noise, and family support at the bedside. Cluster activities to allow for uninterrupted periods of sleep or "sleep hours."

Assess pain on 0–10 scale or faces scale and look for nonverbal cues. See Agitation, Sedation, and Pain Assessment Scales.

Medications for Agitation, Sedation, and Pain

Benzodiazepines

- Diazepam (Valium)
- Lorazepam (Ativan)
- Midazolam (Versed)
- Frequently combined with opioids. Use caution in elderly patients
- Keep flumazenil (Romazicon) available (a benzodiazepine antagonist/antidote)

Opioids

- Morphine sulfate
- Fentanyl
- Hydromorphone (Dilaudid)
- Consider oxycodone (OxyContin) as needed
- Consider remifentanil (Ultiva) as needed

Nonopioid Analgesics
- Ketamine

Alpha-Adrenergic Receptor Agonists
- Dexmedetomidine (Precedex)

Nonbarbiturate Sedatives
- Propofol (Diprivan)
- Etomidate (Amidate)

Physiological Responses to Pain and Anxiety

- Tachycardia
- Diaphoresis
- Sleep disturbance
- Hypertension
- Tachypnea
- Nausea

Signs of Sedative or Analgesic Withdrawal
- Nausea, vomiting, diarrhea
- Cramps, muscle aches
- Increased sensitivity to pain
- Tachypnea, ↑ HR, ↑ BP
- Delirium, tremors, seizures, agitation

Medication Management

- Administer analgesics as scheduled doses or continuous infusions; avoid prn analgesics.
- Other routes include oral, rectal, transdermal, subcutaneous, and spinal.
- Opioids preferred: fentanyl, hydromorphone, and morphine.
- Have naloxone (Narcan), an opioid antagonist, available.
- Monitor body and limb movements, facial expression, posturing, muscle tension for signs of pain.
- Monitor for acute changes or fluctuations in mental status, LOC, disorientation, hallucinations, delusions.
- Evaluate arousability.
- Monitor neurological status including pupillary response, response to verbal commands and pain.
- Monitor respiratory rate and respiratory effort, respiratory depression, BP, HR.

Agitation, Sedation, and Pain Assessment Scales

Richmond Agitation Sedation Scale (RASS)

Score	Term	Description
+4	Combative	Overtly combative, violent, immediate danger to staff
+3	Very agitated	Pulls or removes tube(s) or catheter(s); aggressive
+2	Agitated	Frequent nonpurposeful movement, fights ventilator
+1	Restless	Anxious but movements not aggressive vigorous
0	Alert and calm	
−1	Drowsy	Not fully alert, but has sustained awakening to verbal stimuli (eye-opening/eye contact) to *voice/verbal stimuli (>10 sec)*
−2	Light sedation	Briefly awakens with eye contact to *voice/verbal stimuli (<10 sec)*
−3	Moderate sedation	Movement or eye opening to voice/verbal *stimuli (but no eye contact)*
−4	Deep sedation	No response to voice, but movement or eye opening to physical stimulation
−5	Unarousable	*No response to voice or physical stimulation*

Procedure for RASS Assessment

Procedure	Patient Assessment	Score
1. Observe patient.	a. Patient is alert, restless, or agitated.	0 to +4
2. If not alert, state patient's name and *say* to open eyes and look at speaker.	b. Patient awakens with sustained eye opening and eye contact.	−1
	c. Patient awakens with eye opening and eye contact, but not sustained.	−2
	d. Patient has any movement in response to voice but no eye contact.	−3

Continued

Procedure for RASS Assessment—cont'd

Procedure	Patient Assessment	Score
3. When no response to verbal stimulation, physically stimulate patient by shaking shoulder and/or rubbing sternum.	e. Patient has any movement to physical stimulation.	−4
	f. Patient has no response to any stimulation.	−5

Reprinted with permission from Vanderbilt University. http://www.icudelirium.org/docs/RASS.pdf.

Sedation-Agitation Scale (SAS)

Score	Level of Sedation-Agitation	Response
7	Dangerous agitation	Pulling at endotracheal tube, thrashing, climbing over bed rails
6	Very agitated	Does not calm, requires restraints, bites endotracheal tube
5	Agitated	Attempts to sit up but calms to verbal instructions
4	Calm and cooperative	Obeys commands
3	Sedated	Difficult to rouse, obeys simple commands
2	Very sedated	Rouses to stimuli; does not obey commands
1	Unarousable	Minimal or no response to noxious stimuli

Reprinted with permission from Riker, R, Fraser, GL, and Cox, PM. Continuous infusion of halo-peridol controls agitation in critically ill patients. Crit Care Med 22(3):433–440, 1994.

BASICS

Pain Assessment Scales

Pain Visual Analog Scale (VAS)

no pain 0	5	worst pain 10
no anxiety		severe anxiety

- Nonverbal Adult Pain Assessment Scale (NVPS)
- Behavioral Pain Scale (BPS)
- Critical Care Pain Observation Tool (CPOT) for nonverbal adults
- Faces Pain Scale

Pain Management

- Continuous IV narcotic
- Patient controlled analgesia
- Epidural analgesia

Delirium

Delirium has been associated with poor patient outcomes. Patients with delirium have higher ICU and hospital stays along with a higher risk of death. Usually reversible. More common in elderly patients, patients with compromised mental status, and mechanically ventilated patients. AACN recommends the THINK mnemonic in determining the cause of delirium in ICU patients:

- **T**oxic situations
  - HF, shock, dehydration
  - Delirogenic meds (tight titration of sedatives)
  - New organ failure (e.g., liver, kidney)
- **H**ypoxemia
- **I**nfection/sepsis (nosocomial)
- **N**onpharmacological interventions (Are these being neglected?)
  - Immobilization
  - Hearing aids, glasses, sleep protocols, music, noise control, ambulation
- **K**$^+$ or electrolyte problems

May also be precipitated by hypertension, head trauma, and metabolic disturbances.

Delirium is characterized by an acute onset of mental status changes that develop over a short period of time, usually hours to days. It may fluctuate over the course of a day. It may be combined with inattention and disorganized thinking or altered level of consciousness. The DSM-IV-TR describes three clinical subtypes: hyperactive, hypoactive, and mixed. Hyperactive delirium may be confused with anxiety and agitation.

Other signs and symptoms include:

- Difficulty maintaining or shifting attention with low attention span.
- Variation in levels of confusion; disorientation; fluctuations between lucidity and confusion.
- Illusions, paranoia, or hallucinations.
- Fluctuating LOC with clouding of consciousness.
- Dysphasia; dysarthria.
- Tremor; motor abnormalities; asterixis if hepatic encephalopathy suspected.
- Benzodiazepines such as lorazepam (Ativan) may cause or worsen delirium and should be avoided. Opioid analgesics, metoclopramide, antidepressants, H_2 antagonists and corticosteroids have also been identified as risk factors for delirium development. Review all of patient's medications that may be causing/exacerbating delirium.
- Newer neuroleptics preferred. Consider risperidone (Risperdal), olanzapine (Zyprexa), and quetiapine (Seroquel). Consider melatonin and remelteon.
- Haloperidol (Haldol) is commonly used to treat delirium in the ICU patient but has shown to have adverse neurological effects. If used, monitor for QT prolongation.

Delirium Assessment Tools

The Confusion Assessment Method for the Intensive Care Unit (CAM-ICU) score is widely used to screen for delirium in the ICU population.

Confusion Assessment Method for the ICU (CAM-ICU) Flowsheet. http://www.icudelirium.org/docs/CAM_ICU_flowsheet.pdf

Confusion Assessment Method for the ICU (CAM-ICU) Worksheet. Refer to: www.icudelirium.org/docs/CAN_ICU_worksheet.pdf

Assessment tools to predict delirium and severity of delirium in hospitalized patients.

- Mini-Cog
- Intensive Care Delirium Severity Checklist (ICDSC)
- Delirium Detection Scale (DDS)

Complications of Sedation, Agitation, and Delirium Therapy

- Hypotension
- Patient unresponsiveness
- Respiratory depression
- Delayed weaning from mechanical ventilator

Complications associated with immobility: pressure ulcers, thromboembolism, gastric ileus, hospital-acquired pneumonia

Management of the Patient With Agitation or Delirium

- Institute delirium protocol. Refer to: http://www.icudelirium.org/docs/Delirium-Protocol.pdf
- Monitor for delirium onset and resolution of symptoms.
- Systematic use of standardized assessment tools should be used. Example: All elderly patients should be screened with the CAM-ICU on ICU admission.
- Provide a quiet and stable environment. Promote rest and control pain.
- Provide reality orientation in any patient encounter.
- Institute safety precautions. Physical restraints should be a last option.
- Monitor VS and pulse oximetry. P/F ratio should improve in ARDS patients.
- Monitor ECG.
- Ensure adequate nutrition.
- Provide progressive mobility exercise.
- Monitor CBC; electrolytes; glucose levels; renal, liver, and thyroid function tests; urinalysis; vitamin B$_{12}$ and thiamine levels; HIV status; urine and blood toxicology; and ETOH levels.
- CT, MRI, ECG, EEG, or CXR may be ordered to rule out physical courses of delirium.
- S-100 calcium-binding protein B (S100B) are seen in higher levels in patients with delirium.
- AACN recommends the ABCDEF bundle (refer to Basics, Mechanical Ventilation).

Medically Induced Coma

Also referred to as barbiturate coma.

Causes a temporary coma or a deep state of unconsciousness to protect the brain from swelling and allow the brain to rest to help prevent brain damage. Goal is to reduce ICP.

Medications used: propofol, pentobarbital, thiopental.

Acute Coronary Syndrome (ACS)

ACS is the term used to denote any one of three clinical manifestations of coronary artery disease:

- Unstable angina
- Non–ST-elevation MI (NSTEMI)
- ST-elevation MI (STEMI)

Pathophysiology

Unstable angina represents the progression of stable coronary artery disease to unstable disease. Rupture of atherosclerotic plaque causes thrombus formation and partial occlusion in coronary arteries that precipitate a myocardial infarction.

Clinical Presentation

ACS manifests with chest pain, diaphoresis, SOB, nausea and vomiting, dyspnea, weakness, fatigue, and exercise intolerance. Symptoms of MI are midsternal chest pain described as pressure, squeezing, fullness, or pain. May radiate to jaw, neck, arms, or back and usually lasts more than 15 min.

Assessment for chest pain and associated symptoms of ACS include use of PQRST method when assessing pain, physical exam, vital signs, auscultation for S_3 or S_4 gallop, auscultation of lungs for crackles, and assessment of peripheral vessels for pulse deficits or bruits.

Diagnostic Tests

- ECG
- Echocardiogram
- Cycle cardiac markers (troponin I, CK, CK-MB, myoglobin, C-reactive protein)
- Chest x-ray
- Nuclear scan
- CT angiography
- Coronary angiogram
- Fibrinogen level
- Homocystine lipoprotein levels
- Total cholesterol and triglyceride levels
- Brain natriuretic peptide (BNP)
- PT/PTT

Management

- Administer oxygen to maintain SaO$_2$ >93%.
- Establish IV access.
- Perform continuous cardiac monitoring.
- Administer SL nitroglycerin tablets or oral spray, every 5 min × 3 doses, if pain persists. IV nitroglycerin may be started.
- Monitor for hypotension and headaches from vasodilatation.
- Administer non–enteric-coated aspirin (162–325 mg) and have patient chew it, if not already on daily dose.
- Administer IV morphine, 4–8 mg initially with increments of 2–8 mg repeated at 5–15 min intervals until pain is controlled. Use lower dose in elderly patients.
- Monitor for hypotension and respiratory depression.
- Unless contraindicated, administer a beta blocker.
- Administer angiotensin converting enzyme inhibitors (ACE-IS) and angiotensin receptor blockers (ARBs) if patient had moderate to severe MI with reduced heart's pumping capacity.
- Administer calcium channel blockers if symptoms persist after NTG and beta blockers given.
- Monitor and immediately treat arrhythmias; pay attention to electrolyte disturbances (especially potassium and magnesium), hypoxemia, drugs, or acidosis.
- Administer clopidogrel 300–600 mg loading dose (600 mg preferred dose).
- High-risk patients with NSTEMI ACS should also receive unfractionated heparin or low-molecular-weight heparin (LMWH) and IV platelet glycoprotein IIb/IIIa complex blockers (tirofiban, eptifibatide), as well as ASA, clopidogrel, and beta blockers.

Unstable Angina

Unstable angina is the sudden onset of chest pain, pressure, or tightness resulting from insufficient blood flow through coronary arteries.

Pathophysiology

Atherosclerosis → obstruction of coronary arteries → decrease blood flow through coronary arteries → decrease oxygen supply to myocardial demand for O$_2$ during exertion or emotional stress → angina.

Clinical Presentation

Chest pain manifests as follows: substernal pain, tightness, dullness, fullness, heaviness, or pressure; dyspnea; sweating; syncope; and pain radiating to arms, epigastrium, shoulder, neck, or jaw. Women may experience more atypical symptoms such as back pain and GI symptoms (e.g., indigestion, nausea and vomiting, and abdominal fullness), whereas men may experience typical symptoms such as midsternal chest pain radiating to the left arm.

Diagnostic Tests

- 12-lead ECG
- Lab work: cardiac markers: creatine kinase (CK), creatine kinase–myocardial band (CK-MB), troponin I (TnI), and myoglobin
- Exercise or pharmacological stress test
- Echocardiogram
- Nuclear scan: single-photon emission computed tomography (SPECT), MRI with gadolinium enhancement (MUGA)
- Cardiac catheterization and coronary artery angiography
- Percutaneous coronary intervention (PCI)
- Chest x-ray
- MRI/MRA, myocardial perfusion imaging
- CBC, CMP, lipid panel, BNP

Management

- Calculate TIMI Risk Score for patients with unstable angina (UA) and non–ST-elevation MI (NSTEMI). Estimates mortality for patients with unstable angina and NSTEMI. Refer to: http://www.mdcalc.com/timi-risk-score-for-uanstemi/
- Ensure bedrest.
- Obtain ECG and lab work.
- Assess chest pain for frequency, duration, cause that triggered pain, radiation of pain, and intensity based on pain scale from 0 to 10, with 0 being no pain and 10 being worst pain.
- Supply O_2.
- Provide continuous cardiac monitoring.
- Pharmacological treatment:
  - Early conservative, for low-risk patient: anti-ischemic, antiplatelet, and antithrombotic drug therapy; stress and treadmill tests.
  - Early invasive: same drug therapy as early conservative but followed by diagnostic catheterization and revascularization.
  - Administer nitroglycerin (NTG): 0.4 mg (SL or spray) every 5 min for a total of three doses → IV infusion start at 5–10 mcg/min, titrate for pain

according to hospital policy. Dose should not exceed 400 mcg/min; check for contraindications such as hypotension, or if taking the following meds: Viagra, Cialis, or Levitra.

- Administer morphine sulfate IV if symptoms persist after receiving NTG or in patients who have pulmonary congestion or severe agitation.
- Administer beta blocker: metoprolol (Lopressor).
- Administer ACE-IS in patients with LV dysfunction or HF with renal HTN; not recommended in patients with renal failure.
- Administer calcium channel blockers: verapamil (Calan, Isoptin) or diltiazem (Cardizem) if patient not responding to beta blocker or nitrates.

Use severe caution when combining blocking agents

- Administer antiplatelet: aspirin 162–325 mg, chewed.
- Administer GP IIb/IIIa inhibitor: abciximab (ReoPro), eptifibatide (Integrilin) or tirofiban (Aggrastat) if no contraindications (i.e., bleeding, stroke in past month, severe HTN, renal dialysis, major surgery within the past 6 wk, or platelet count <100,000 mm³).
- Administer antithrombotic: heparin.
- Administer anticoagulant: enoxaparin (Lovenox).
- Administer clopidogrel (Plavix).
- Administer direct thrombin inhibitor (hirudin, bivalirudin).

Acute Myocardial Infarction (AMI)

AMI is the acute death of myocardial cells resulting from lack of oxygenated blood flow in the coronary arteries. It is also known as a heart attack.

Pathophysiology

Injury to the artery's endothelium → increases platelet adhesion → inflammatory response causing monocytes and T lymphocytes to migrate in the intima → macrophages and smooth muscle distend with lipids, to form fatty streaks and a fibrous cap → thinning of cap increases susceptibility to rupture or hemorrhage → rupture triggers thrombus formation and vasoconstriction → result: thrombus with narrowing artery. If occlusion lasts more than 20 min, can lead to AMI.

Clinical Presentation

AMI manifests with chest pain or discomfort lasting 20 min or longer. Pain can be described as pressure, tightness, heaviness, burning, or a squeezing or crushing sensation, located typically in the central chest or epigastrium; it may radiate to the arms, shoulders, neck, jaw, or back.

Discomfort may be accompanied by weakness, dyspnea, diaphoresis, or anxiety; not relieved by NTG. Women may experience atypical discomfort, SOB, or fatigue. Diabetic patients may not display classic signs and symptoms of AMI. Elderly patients may experience SOB, pulmonary edema, dizziness, altered mental status.

ST-segment elevation MI: Look for tall positive T waves and ST-segment elevation of 1 mm or more above baseline.

Non–ST-segment elevation MI: May include ST-segment depression and T-wave inversion.

Diagnostic Tests

- ECG findings.
- Cardiac markers (CK, myoglobin, and troponins).
- Ischemia modified albumin (IMA): measures changes in serum albumin when in contact with ischemic tissue. IMA rises faster than other cardiac enzymes.
- Serum cardiac biomarkers; timeline varies according to reference.

Biomarker	Levels Increase	Levels Peak	Remain Elevated for
CK	3–6 hr	24–36 hr	3–5 days
CK-MB	3–8 hr after chest pain onset	12–24 hr	48–72 hr
Myoglobin	30 min–4 hr after chest pain onset	6–12 hr	24–36 hr
Troponin	Within 3–12 hr after MI	14–48 hr	5–14 days
Troponin I	Within 3–12 hr	14–24 hr	5–14 days
Troponin T	Within 3–12 hr	12–48 hr	5–14 days
IMA	Within 2 min of MI	6 hr	12 hr

- Echocardiogram.
- PCI.

Management

Management is based on the 2013 ACCF/AHA Guideline for the Management of ST-Elevation Myocardial Infarction.

- Calculate TIMI Risk Score for ST Elevation MI (STEMI). Estimates mortality in patients with STEMI. Refer to: http://www.mdcalc.com/timi-risk-score-for-stemi/

- Calculate the HEART Score, a tool for predicting and managing the risk of heart attack and stroke. Refer to: https://www.mdcalc.com/heart-score-major-cardiac-events
- Calculate in-hospital and 6-mo mortality rate for patients with ACS including those with ST elevation or ST depression using the Global Registry of Acute Coronary Events (GRACE) risk model. Refer to: http://www.outcomes-umassmed.org/grace/acs_risk/acs_risk_content.html
- Focus on pain radiation, SOB, and diaphoresis.
- Obtain a 12-lead ECG and lab draw for cardiac markers.
- MONA: morphine, O_2, NTG, and 162-325 mg non-enteric coated aspirin po or chewed. If allergic to aspirin, give ticlopidine (Ticlid) or clopidogrel (Plavix).
- Administer supplemental O_2 to maintain SpO_2 >90%.
- Administer sublingual NTG tablets or spray.
- Administer IV morphine 2-8 mg initially and then 2-8 mg every 5-15 min until pain is controlled. (Monitor for hypotension and respiratory depression).
- Administer ACE-Is or ARBs.
- Administer statin.
- Administer beta blocker.
- Administer unfractionated heparin, low-molecular-weight heparin.
- Administer glycoprotein IIb/IIIa antagonists (abciximab, eptifibatide, tirofiban).
- Coronary arterial bypass graft (CABG) is warranted in setting of failed PCI with instability.

ST-Segment Monitoring

- Continuous ST-segment monitoring is used to detect silent ischemia in asymptomatic select patients. Monitoring ST changes in a 12-lead ECG is most accurate. If continuous 12-lead ECG not available, use leads III and V_3.
- Be sure to select patient's most sensitive monitoring leads (ST fingerprint).
- Evaluate ST segment with patient in supine position (change in body position can alter ST segment and mimic ischemia). If ST alarm sounds with patient in side-lying position, return patient to supine. If deviation persists in supine, may indicate ischemia.
- Measure the ST-segment changes 60 msec beyond the J point (the junction of the QRS complex with the ST segment).
- Alarm parameters:
  - Patients at high risk for ischemia: Set ST-segment alarm parameters 1 mm above and below baseline ST segment.
  - Stable patients: Set segment alarm parameters 2 mm above and below baseline ST segment.

- Document actual millimeters of ST-segment depression or elevation.
- Cause for concern: ST depression or elevation of 1–2 mm that lasts for at least 1 min can be clinically significant and warrants further patient assessments.

Hypertensive Urgency and Emergency

- **Hypertensive emergency**: Rapid (hours to days) marked elevation in BP (SBP >180 mm Hg or DBP >120 mm Hg) → acute organ tissue damage.
- **Hypertensive urgency**: Slow (days to weeks) elevation in BP (SBP >180 mm Hg or DBP >110 mm Hg) usually does not lead to organ tissue damage.

Pathophysiology

Any disorder or cause (essential hypertension, renal parenchymal disease, renovascular disease, pregnancy, endocrine drugs, autonomic hyperreactivity, CNS disorder) → ↑ BP → vessel becomes inflamed → leak fluid or blood to the brain → CVA → long-term disability. Intense vasoconstriction may also cause encephalopathy, myocardial ischemia or infarction, acute pulmonary edema, aortic dissection, and acute renal failure, among other conditions.

Clinical Presentation

Hypertensive crisis manifests with:

- Chest pain
- Dyspnea, orthopnea, paroxysmal nocturnal dyspnea
- Neurological deficits
- Severe, throbbing headache
- Visual disturbances
- Nausea and vomiting
- Dysphagia
- Back pain
- Severe anxiety
- Irritability, confusion
- Possible seizures
- Oliguria if kidneys affected

Diagnostic Tests

- CT or MRI of chest, abdomen, and brain
- 2-D echocardiogram or transesophageal echocardiogram
- ECG
- CBC
- Cardiac biomarkers if appropriate
- Serum BUN, creatinine, BMP
- Urinalysis especially gravity, urine toxicology
- Renal ultrasound if kidney involvement
- Chest x-ray (if dyspnea or chest pain present)

Management

- Administer O₂ to maintain Pao₂ >92%. Monitor ABGs.
- Obtain VS: orthostatic BP every 5 min, then longer intervals. Arterial line recommended.
- Check BP in both arms.
- Palpate pulses in all extremities.
- Provide continuous ECG monitoring and treatment of arrhythmias.
- Assess cardiac, respiratory, and neurological status.
- Administer sodium nitroprusside (Nipride) but titrate carefully for acute drop in BP. Monitor for thiocyanate and cyanide toxicity.
- Administer analgesics for pain or headache.
- Administer labetalol (Trandate) or esmolol (Brevibloc) if hypertensive encephalopathy present.
- Consider fenoldopam (Corlopam), clevidipine (Cleviprex), or enalapril (Vasotec). Also consider the use of nitroglycerine (NTG).
- Propranolol (Inderal) is not recommended for hypertensive crisis.
- Hypertensive emergency: IV route is preferred; reduce mean arterial pressure (MAP) by no more than 25% in the first hour; if stable, ↓ diastolic BP to 100–110 mm Hg over the next 2–6 hr.
- If neurological complication develops, primary goal → maintain adequate cerebral perfusion; control HTN, minimize cerebral edema; ↓ BP by 10% but no more than 20%–30% from initial reading.
- Hypertensive urgency: Give po meds: ↓ BP in 24-48 hr; use short-acting agents: captopril (Capoten) or clonidine (Catapres).
- Provide a quiet environment with low lighting. Cluster activities to provide rest and sleep.

Heart Failure (HF)

HF, which is sometimes referred to as "pump failure," is a general term for the inadequacy of the heart to pump blood throughout the body. This deficit causes insufficient perfusion to body tissues with vital nutrients and oxygen.

Pathophysiology

HF failure can be classified into left-sided failure and right-sided failure. Both may be acute or chronic and mild to severe, caused by HTN, CAD, or valvular disease, involving the mitral or aortic valve. HF can also be divided into two subtypes: systolic heart failure and diastolic heart failure.

- Systolic heart failure results when the heart is unable to contract forcefully enough, during systole, to eject adequate amounts of blood into the circulation. Preload increases with decreased contractility, and afterload increases as a result of increased peripheral resistance.
- Diastolic heart failure occurs when the left ventricle is unable to relax adequately during diastole. Inadequate relaxation prevents the ventricle from filling with sufficient blood to ensure adequate cardiac output.

Clinical Presentation

Left-sided HF manifests as:

- Dyspnea, SOB, orthopnea, paroxysmal nocturnal dyspnea
- Nonproductive cough
- Diaphoresis
- Chest pain, pressure or palpitations
- Tachycardia, which may be weak and thready
- S_3 gallop
- Tachypnea
- Pulmonary crackles or wheezes
- JVD
- Frothy, pink-tinged sputum; hemoptysis; pulmonary edema
- Central or peripheral cyanosis or pallor
- Fatigue, weakness
- Confusion, restlessness

Right-sided HF manifests as:

- Right upper quadrant pain
- Peripheral edema, initially dependent then pitting. Weight gain
- JVD
- Hepatomegaly, hepatojugular reflux

- Ascites or anasarca
- Nocturia
- HTN
- Anorexia, nausea

Diagnostic Tests

- B-type natriuretic peptide (BNP) level
- CBC
- BMP, lipid profile, iron studies, renal and liver function tests
- TSH levels
- Urinalysis
- Chest x-ray
- ABGs or pulse oximetry, Pulmonary function tests
- ECG
- 2-D echocardiogram
- MUGA scan
- Hemodynamic studies using a PAP catheter
- Stress test (noninvasive) if possible

Management

The following serves only as a guide to the treatment of heart failure. For a full discussion and criteria for the administration of medications, refer to the 2017 American College of Cardiology Foundation/American Heart Association Guideline for the Management of Heart Failure at http://circ.aha-journals.org/content/circulationaha/early/2017/04/26/CIR.0000000000000509.full.pdf?utm_medium=referral&utm_source=r360

- Primary goal in managing heart failure is to maintain cardiac output.
- Secondary goal is to decrease venous (capillary) pressure to limit edema.
- Monitor cardiac, respiratory, renal, and neurological status.
- Place patient in Fowler's position.
- Administer O_2 via cannula or mask. Intubate if necessary. Consider noninvasive positive pressure ventilation first.
- Monitor O_2 saturation.
- Provide continuous ECG monitoring.
- Monitor hemodynamic status.
- Weigh daily. Assess edema.
- Provide sodium and fluid restrictions.
- Assess fluid and electrolyte balance.
- Provide maximum rest. Cluster activities.
- Administer diuretics to control edema and fluid retention: furosemide (Lasix), bumetanide (Bumex), torsemide (Demadex).

- In patients not responsive to loop diuretics, administer hydrochlorothiazide (Microzide), indapamide, chlorthalidone (Thalitone), chlorothiazide (Diuril), metolazone (Zaroxolyn), spironolactone (Aldactone), amiloride (Midamor), or triamterene (Dyrenium).
- Consider low-dose dopamine to support renal function.
- Administer beta blockers to reduce cardiac workload, improve LV ejection fraction, and prevent arrhythmias: metoprolol (Lopressor, Toprol XL), carvedilol (Coreg), or bisoprolol (Zebeta).
- Administer nitrates to enhance myocardial contractility and decrease LV filling pressure and SVR: NTG, isosorbide, nitroprusside.
- Administer inotropes to enhance myocardial contractility and increase organ perfusion: dopamine, dobutamine, milrinone, and digoxin (Lanoxin).
- Administer ACE-IS to reduce peripheral resistance, afterload, preload, and heart size: captopril enalapril (Vasotec), lisinopril (Prinivil), ramipril (Altace) or quinapril (Accupril).
- Administer angiotensin II receptor blockers to reduce afterload: losartan (Cozaar), valsartan (Diovan), candesartan (Atacand), irbesartan (Avapro), azilsartan (Edarbi).
- Administer vasodilators if adequate BP to decrease preload and/or afterload and SVR: nitroprusside (Nitropress) or hydralazine.
- Administer nesiritide (Natrecor) to reduce PCWP and improve dyspnea.
- Administer alpha-beta-adrenergic agonists to improve cardiac output and organ perfusion: epinephrine or norepinephrine (Levophed).
- Consider aldosterone antagonists in select cases: eplerenone (Inspra).
- Administer anticoagulants to prevent thromboembolism: warfarin (Coumadin), dabigatran (Pradaxa), or rivaroxaban (Xarelto). Monitor closely for signs of bleeding.
- Consider sildenafil (Viagra) in select instances.
- Administer morphine for pain.
- Avoid NSAIDs and calcium channel blockers as they can exacerbate HF. Many antiarrhythmics are also contraindicated in HF.
- Prepare patient for biventricular pacemaker or AICD.
- Other procedures that may be necessary include:
    - Ultrafiltration for patients who have significant volume overload unresponsive to diuretics
    - Coronary artery bypass graft (CABG) or percutaneous coronary intervention (PCI)
    - Valvular surgery on the aortic or mitral valve
    - Cardiac resynchronization therapy (CRT)
    - Ventricular restoration procedures
    - Extracorporeal membrane oxygenator (ECMO)
    - Ventricular assist device (VAD)
    - Heart transplant

Ventricular Assist Devices (VADs)

- VADs are used in the treatment of acute or chronic heart failure refractory to standard treatment and a failing heart. Supports the left ventricle (LVAD), the right ventricle (RVAD), or both ventricles (BIVAD). They improve end-organ function, quality of life, and extend survival. May be used short or long term and implanted internally or located externally.
- The devices are also categorized as pulsatile or nonpulsatile (newer pumps, continuous flow).
  - Continuous flow pump: Nonpulsatile; continuously fills and returns blood to a major blood vessel at a constant preset rate.
  - Pulsatile flow pump: Fills during systole and pumps blood into aorta during diastole or pulmonary artery or may pump regardless of the patient's (native) cardiac cycle.
- All devices use the same concept. Blood is removed from the failing ventricle and is diverted into a pump that delivers blood to the aorta (in the case of the LVAD) or the pulmonary artery (in the case of the RVAD).
- LVADs can often be placed temporarily and serve as a bridge to recovery in patients with acute, severe cardioveritis or post cardiotomy. In patients with end-stage heart failure, VADs are a bridge to heart transplantation that allows some patients to undergo rehabilitation and possibly go home before transplantation.
- Long-term use may be considered when no definitive procedure is planned, and lifelong use may be considered if patient is not a candidate or does not want cardiac transplantation.

Procedure:

- Done under general anesthesia; a sternotomy is performed. A "pericardial cradle" is created with sutures to lift the heart up for better visualization of the heart structures.
- A pump pocket is then created to make a space for the device to sit in (extraperitoneal), an area below the rectus abdominis and internal oblique muscles and above the posterior rectus sheath, or intraperitoneal).
- After the pocket is prepared and the patient is cannulated, cardiopulmonary bypass is initiated. An inflow cannula is placed in the LV apex and secured with sutures.
- The pump is placed in the abdominal pocket, the length of the outflow graft is measured (should lie under the right sternal border), and the driveline (a tunneling device) is performed. This is done by placement through a skin incision to the right of the umbilicus and tunneled to the device pocket.
- The outflow cannula is placed, then de-aired; the patient is weaned from cardiopulmonary bypass, and the device is activated.

Management

Routine postoperative care with special attention to the following:

- Assess lung sounds, respirations, and O_2 saturation and ABGs. Pulse oximetry unreliable.
- Keep intubated until anesthesia cleared from system.
- Assess cardiac sounds, rate, rhythm. Continuous ECG monitoring. Pacing with epicardial wires may be warranted.
- A VAD-generated pulse and patient's intrinsic or native electrical activity will both appear on the monitoring system. The VAD-generated pulse is ordered in a fixed-rate mode or volume or automatic mode.
- If VF or asystole occurs, patient will still have a palpable pulse resulting from ongoing pump ejection of the VAD.
- Assess neurological status to ensure cerebral perfusion.
- Monitor VS. Administer vasodilators as needed for MAP 65–80/90 mm Hg. Automated BP cuffs unreliable. Use arterial line. BP measurement via Doppler recommended if no A-line.
- Monitor hemodynamics: cardiac index, cardiac output, CVP, PAP, PCWP.
- Monitor fluid and electrolyte balance including urine output. Note signs of fluid overload and decreased urinary output.
- Administer anticoagulants (unfractionated heparin, warfarin, aspirin).
- Assess incisions and dressings for drainage, bleeding, erythema.
- Obtain and monitor labs: CMP, CBC, PT/PTT, with close attention to K^+ and Mg.
- Medicate for pain as needed.
- Antibiotics may be ordered prophylactically.
- The patient is also monitored via chest x-rays and echocardiograms.
- Address psychosocial issues and refer as needed.

Complications

- Device malfunction resulting from mechanical problems or thrombosis
- Infection
- Low flow or output of the VAD
- Pulmonary embolism or stroke
- Cardiac arrhythmias
- RV dysfunction in left VAD implantation
- Hemorrhage, cardiac tamponade
- Secondary organ dysfunction including kidneys, liver, lungs, and brain

Abdominal Aortic Aneurysm (AAA)

AAA is a localized, chronic abnormal dilation of an artery located between the renal and iliac arteries with a diameter at least 1.5 times that of the expected diameter and a natural history toward enlargement and rupture.

Pathophysiology

Atherosclerosis and destruction of elastin and collagen fibers in the vessel walls contribute to its development.

Pathophysiology for Atherosclerosis

Fatty streaks deposited in arterial intima → stimulates inflammatory response that causes proliferation → proliferation causes blood vessel to form fibrous capillaries → deposits build up as atheromas or plaques ← plaques pile up, obstructing the blood flow → outpouching of abdominal aneurysm.

Pathophysiology Involvement With Elastin and Collagen

Media thins → decrease in elastin fibers in vessel walls ← collagen weakens ← leads to aneurysm growth → outpouching of abdominal aorta.

Clinical Presentation

AAA may manifest as asymptomatic or symptomatic. When asymptomatic, look for a pulsatile, periumbilical mass with or without a bruit. When symptomatic, symptoms include:

- Sudden, severe constant pain in the abdomen, flank, groin, or back
- Early satiety, gastric or abdominal fullness, nausea and vomiting, GI bleeding
- Syncope
- Unequal carotid pulses and different BP in right and left arms
- ↑ peripheral circulation, venous thrombosis, lower extremity ischemia
- Pulsatile mass may be felt in abdomen
- Symptoms of shock with rupture

AAA can also mimic:

- Urinary tract infection or kidney infection
- Renal calculus or obstruction
- Ruptured disc
- Diverticulitis or ischemic bowel
- Pancreatitis
- Incarcerated hernia

- Abdominal neoplasm
- Peptic ulcer perforation, GI bleed

Diagnostic Tests

- CBC with differential, metabolic panel
- Abdominal ultrasound (first line of diagnostic testing)
- CT scan of the abdomen
- Abdominal x-ray
- Echocardiogram may be useful
- Aortogram
- MRI
- Preoperative labs and type and crossmatch for surgery

Management

- Administer beta blocker to lower arterial pressure to the lowest SBP (120 mm Hg or less). Use alpha-beta blocker labetalol (Trandate) or metoprolol (Lopressor) in place of nitroprusside and a beta blocker; do not give direct vasodilators such as hydralazine.
- Monitoring of oxygenation and ECG.
- If aneurysm ruptures:
  - Administer IV propranolol (Inderal) to ↓ myocardial contractility and keep HR 60–80 bpm.
  - Administer nitroprusside to maintain MAP 70–80 mm Hg.
  - Provide fluid resuscitation.
  - Administer morphine for pain.
  - Prepare patient for emergency surgery.

Postoperative Management

- Goal of postoperative care is to reduce afterload and pressure at the repair site.
- Administer IV nitroprusside with esmolol (Brevibloc) or labetalol (Trandate) and titrate the dosage to keep systolic BP below 120 mm Hg as ordered.
- Starting immediately after surgery, continuously monitor the patient's neurological status, cardiac rhythm, RR, hemodynamics, urine output, core body temperature, fluid and electrolyte imbalance.
- Provide analgesia. Morphine recommended.
- Monitor for acute renal failure, ischemic colitis, spinal cord ischemia, and aortoenteric fistula.
- Assess patient's gastrointestinal function.
- Report urine output less than 0.5 mL/kg/hr, which indicates dehydration, volume deficit, or decreased renal function.

- Anticoagulants may be needed to prevent thrombi formation.
- Assess for poor peripheral perfusion.

Aortic Dissection

Aortic dissection is a tear (without hematoma or an intramural hematoma) in the aortic wall that causes a longitudinal separation between the intima and adventitia layers resulting in diversion of blood flow from its normal arterial pathway. Aortic dissection requires emergency surgery.

Pathophysiology

Tear in aorta intima → blood flows into subintimal region → pulsatile pressure creates a false channel between intimal and medial layers of aorta → intimal and medial layer is separated → circulatory volume decreases → channel expands and creates either an expanding mass or a hematoma (from blood coagulating) → lumen narrows and obstructs blood flow, cardiac output decreases → results in end-organ failure, also diverted blood can pool around heart, resulting in cardiac tamponade.

Clinical Presentation

Consider acute phase if diagnosed within first 2 wk of onset of pain.

Presenting Symptoms
- Mimics inferior wall MI
- Standard type A aortic dissection: severe chest pain, sometimes sharp
- Standard type B dissection: sudden, severe chest pain radiating to the back; described as "ripping or tearing" pain
- Pain can shift to the abdomen
- Increasing restlessness (sign of extending dissection)
- Decrease in urine output
- Anxiety: "feeling of doom"
- Fainting or dizziness
- Clammy skin
- Nausea and vomiting
- Pallor
- Tachycardia, shortness of breath, orthopnea
- Altered mental status and CVA-type symptoms

Diagnostic Tests

- Chest x-ray: shows widening mediastinum
- ECG
- Transthoracic echocardiogram
- Transesophageal echocardiogram
- CT scan
- Aortic angiography
- MRI
- Doppler imaging
- Cardiac biomarkers if coronary ischemia suspected
- Routine preoperative blood work if surgery anticipated

Management

- The goals of therapy are to control BP and manage pain.
- Measure BP in both arms. Insert arterial line if indicated. Monitor HR, RR, and pain level.
- Perform frequent peripheral pulse checks, ankle brachial index measurements, and neurological assessments.
- Administer beta blockers as first line of treatment; if hypertensive → give nitroprusside IV.
- Labetalol recommended in aortic dissection associated with cocaine ingestion.
- Administer analgesics for pain as appropriate.
- Plan for emergency surgery.

Pericardial Effusion

Pericardial effusion is the abnormal accumulation of more than 50 mL of fluid (normal: 15–50 mL to serve as lubricant for the visceral and parietal layers of pericardium) in the pericardial sac that may lead to noncompression of the heart, which interferes with heart function.

Pathophysiology

Causes: chest trauma, accidents, stab wounds, gunshot wounds, rupture of tumors, obstruction of lymphatic or venous flow, pericarditis, viral infections, cancer, MI, uremia, autoimmune diseases (lupus, rheumatoid arthritis, and others), bacterial infections, or idiopathic → accumulate blood in the pericardial sac → ↑ pressure → compresses or does not compress the heart. May progress to cardiac tamponade.

Clinical Manifestations

Pericardial effusion can be asymptomatic with up to 2 L accumulated fluid in the pericardial sac. Pericardial effusions caused by pericarditis manifest with its main symptom of chest pain; chest pain may be worsened by deep breathing and lessened by leaning forward. If pericarditis is not the cause, there are often no symptoms.

- Complaints of dull, constant pain, pressure, ache, or discomfort in the left side of the chest with symptoms of cardiac compression
- Fever
- Fatigue
- Muscle aches
- Cough, SOB, dyspnea, hoarseness, hiccups
- Nausea, vomiting, and/or diarrhea
- Tachycardia, palpitations
- Light-headedness, syncope
- Cool, clammy skin
- Weakened peripheral pulses, edema, cyanosis
- Anxiety, confusion
- Muffled heart sounds
- May or may not manifest with pericardial friction
- Dullness of percussion of the left lung over the angle of scapula (Ewart's sign)
- ECG showing ↑ voltage of complexes, diffuse ST elevation with PR depression

Diagnostic Tests

- Echocardiogram
- ECG
- Chest x-ray
- CBC with differential, ESR, CRP
- Serum electrolytes
- Blood cultures and cardiac biomarkers as appropriate

Management

- Manage pain.
- Pericardiocentesis or pericardectomy (pericardial window) is performed by a physician.
- Position changes decrease SOB.
- Provide wound care after pericardiocentesis, pericardectomy, or other pericardial surgical procedures, care of pericardial catheters and chest tubes.

- Assess VS, pulses, LOC, respiratory status, skin and temperature changes, intake and output frequently.
- Monitor and record any drainage from pericardial catheters and chest tubes. Refer to Respiratory Tab.
- Depending on etiology of effusion, administer NSAIDs or antibiotics.

Cardiac Surgeries

Coronary Artery Bypass Graft (CABG)

CABG is an open-heart surgical procedure in which a blood vessel from another part of the body, usually the saphenous vein from the leg, is grafted below the occluded coronary artery so that blood can bypass the blockage. CABG may be done with the use of a bypass machine (on pump) or without the use of the machine (off-pump CABG).

Pathophysiology
Surgery is performed on patients with coronary artery disease that causes blockage to the coronary arteries. Fatty streaks deposited in arterial intima stimulate an inflammatory response that causes proliferation. Proliferation causes blood vessels to form fibrous caps, and deposits build up as atheromas or plaques. Plaques pile up, obstructing the blood flow.

Clinical Manifestations
Ischemia: If ischemic episode lasts long enough can cause death to myocardial cells → MI, angina, chest pain, somatic and visceral pain, and discomfort. Atrial fibrillation a common complication of cardiac surgery.

Diagnostic Tests
- Health history
- Routine preoperative lab work including lipid profile, clotting profiles, liver function tests
- Type and crossmatch for blood
- Chest x-ray
- ECG
- Exercise treadmill testing
- Gated SPECT imaging
- Coronary angiography
- Echocardiography
- Electron beam computed tomography (EBCT)

Postoperative Care
- Common post-op care includes maintaining airway patency and monitoring the patient's pulmonary status, vital signs, and intake and output.
- Perform peripheral and neurovascular assessments hourly for first 8 hr.

CV

- Monitor neurological status.
- Monitor cardiac status. Provide continuous ECG monitoring. Treat arrhythmias.
- Monitor hemodynamics. Titrate drugs: vasopressor and inotropes to optimize cardiac function and BP.
- Monitor respiratory status including O_2 saturation and ABGs. Patients are mechanically ventilated on arrival at the ICU.
- Monitor chest tube drainage and record amount.
- Monitor glucose levels and administer insulin as needed.
- Provide DVT and stress ulcer prophylaxis.
- Watch for signs of bleeding, and monitor hemoglobin and hematocrit every 4 hr.
- Monitor patient's pain, and medicate as needed.
- Prevent sternal wound infections.

Complications

- Complications are associated with anesthesia, cardiopulmonary bypass, sternotomy, and the operation itself. These complications may include the following:
  - Myocardial dysfunction including hemodynamic instability
  - Aortic dissection
  - Cardiac tamponade
  - Cerebrovascular complications
  - Acute renal failure
  - Respiratory tract infections; sternal wound infections

Variations of On-Pump CABG

- Off-pump CABG
- Totally endoscopic coronary artery bypass graft
- Minimally invasive direct coronary artery bypass (MIDCAB): small incision made in left chest; internal mammary gland artery sewn to left anterior descending artery

Coronary Stenting/Percutaneous Coronary Intervention (PCI)

PCI is a common intervention for angina, obstructive CAD, myocardial ischemia, prevention of myocardial necrosis, and a nonsurgical alternative to CABG. In a catheterization lab, a catheter equipped with an inflatable balloon tip is inserted into the appropriate coronary artery. When the lesion is located, the catheter is passed through the lesion, the balloon is inflated, and the atherosclerotic plaque is compressed, resulting in vessel dilation. Intracoronary stents are usually inserted during PCI. Stents are used to treat abrupt or threatened abrupt closure or restenosis following PCI.

Procedure

Stents are expandable mesh-like structures designed to maintain vessel patency by compressing the arterial walls and resisting vasoconstriction. Stents are carefully placed over the angioplasty site to hold the vessel open.

Clinical Presentation Prior to PCI

- Atypical or typical chest pain
- SOB
- Dyspnea
- Symptoms of angina or CAD

Diagnostic Tests Prior to PCI

- ECG
- Echocardiogram
- Chest x-ray
- Lab tests: cardiac markers, serum electrolytes, coagulation studies, BUN, creatinine, CBC

Management Post PCI

- Administer antiplatelet agents (aspirin, ticlopidine, clopidogrel).
- Administer IV infusion of glycoprotein IIb/IIIa inhibitors (eptifibatide).
- Monitor for signs and symptoms of bleeding at catheter site.
- Maintain pressure dressing to insertion site for 12 hr after procedure.
- Keep the involved leg straight.
- Set HOB to 45° or less.
- Monitor for cardiac arrhythmias.
- Monitor for chest pain and report immediately to MD. Give O_2, NTG, isosorbide (Imdur), or nifedipine (Procardia); obtain 12-lead ECG.

Complications

- Abrupt closure of dilated segment or stent thrombosis
- Angina, MI, vasospasm, coronary artery dissection

Other interventional cardiology techniques include:

- Laser angioplasty
- Atherectomy, directional coronary atherectomy
- Rotational ablation
- Brachytherapy

Stent Insertion

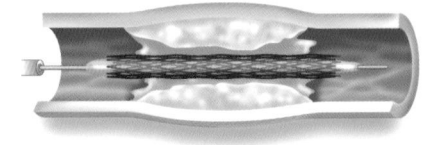

Stent Inflation and Expansion

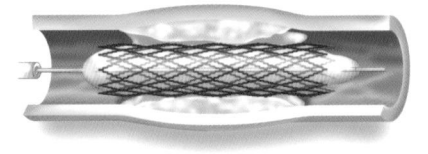

Balloon Removal and Stent Implantation

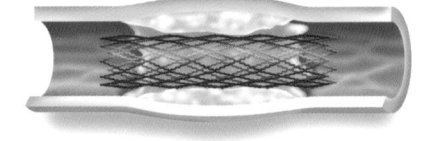

Cardiac Valve Replacement

Clinical conditions that require a surgical procedure to replace the valve with either a mechanical valve or a porcine valve include:

- Acquired valvular dysfunction
- Mitral valve stenosis
- Mitral valve regurgitation
- Mitral valve prolapse
- Aortic stenosis
- Aortic regurgitation
- Pulmonary stenosis (less common)

In some cases of damaged aortic valves, the patients' own pulmonary valve can be used to replace the aortic valve, and then the pulmonary valve is replaced with an artificial valve (the Roth procedure). This is ideal for people who cannot or will not take blood thinners for the rest of their life. The surgical procedure is the same as open-heart surgery except the heart is not bypassed, only the valve is replaced, or it can be minimally invasive; techniques include laparoscopic or endoscopic robot-assisted and percutaneous surgery.

Pathophysiology

- Mitral stenosis: Usually results from rheumatic fever (which can cause valve thickening), atrial myxoma (tumor), calcium accumulation, or thrombus formation → valve becomes stiff. The valve opening narrows → prevention of normal blood flow from left atrium to left ventricle → pulmonary congestion → right-sided heart failure.
- Mitral valve regurgitation: Fibrotic and calcific changes prevent mitral valve from closing completely during systole → incomplete closure of the valve → backflow of blood into left atrium when left ventricle contracts → increased volume ejection with next systole → increased pressure → left ventricular hypertrophy.
- Mitral valve prolapse: The valvular leaflets enlarge and prolapse into left atrium during systole → usually benign but may lead to mitral valve regurgitation.
- Aortic stenosis: Aortic valve orifice narrows and obstructs left ventricle outflow during systole → increased resistance to ejection or afterload → ventricular hypertrophy.
- Aortic regurgitation: Aortic valve leaflets do not close properly → regurgitation of aortic blood back into ventricle during diastole → left ventricular hypertrophy.

Clinical Presentation

- Mitral stenosis: Fatigue, dyspnea on exertion, heart palpitations, heavy coughing, frequent respiratory infections, orthopnea, paroxysmal nocturnal dyspnea, hemoptysis, hepatomegaly, JVD, pitting edema, atrial fibrillation, apical diastolic murmur
- Mitral valve regurgitation: Fatigue, dyspnea on exertion, orthopnea, palpitations, atrial fibrillation, JVD, pitting edema, high-pitched holosystolic murmur

- Mitral valve prolapse: Atypical chest pain, dizziness, syncope, palpitations, atrial tachycardia, ventricular tachycardia, systolic click
- Aortic stenosis: Dyspnea on exertion, angina, syncope on exertion, fatigue, orthopnea, paroxysmal nocturnal dyspnea, harsh systolic crescendo-decrescendo murmur
- Aortic insufficiency: Palpitations, dyspnea, orthopnea, paroxysmal nocturnal dyspnea, fatigue, angina, sinus tachycardia, blowing decrescendo diastolic murmur

Diagnostic Tests

- Echocardiogram
- ECG
- Cardiac angiogram
- Exercise tolerance test
- Chest x-ray

Management

- Routine postoperative care: Maintain airway patency; monitor pulmonary status
- Monitor vital signs and intake and output.
- Perform peripheral and neurovascular assessments hourly for first 8 hr after surgery.
- Monitor dressing and incision for drainage, erythema.
- Monitor neurological status for first 8 hr postoperatively.
- Titrate medications, vasopressors, and inotropes to optimize cardiac function and BP.
- Monitor chest tube drainage.
- Watch for signs of bleeding by monitoring Hgb and Hct every 4 hr.
- Monitor for pain.
- Start on anticoagulation therapy when approved by cardiac surgeon.

Transcatheter Aortic Valve Replacement (TAVR)

- TAVR was developed for the treatment of severe, symptomatic aortic stenosis, for patients at very high surgical risk for traditional valve replacement surgery, or for patients with technical issues with surgery (i.e, porcelain aorta or significant mediastinal radiation).
- Bilateral femoral arteries are prepped, the femoral artery is cannulated with a sheath, and the vessel is dilated. The sheath is replaced by a larger sheath, which is used to accommodate the stent-valve delivery system. An arterial catheter is placed in the left femoral artery for hemodynamic monitoring.

- A guide wire and valvuloplasty balloon catheter are used to steer and deploy the stent-valve. Aortic balloon valvuloplasty is performed to separate the leaflets. Contrast is injected, and fluoroscopy is used to visualize the stent placement.
- When the position of the stent-valve is confirmed, the device is then deployed. Rapid right ventricular pacing reduces cardiac wall motion and prevents the stent-valve from slipping from the correct position during balloon inflation. A temporary pacing lead is placed in the right ventricle via the femoral vein, and temporary pacing is initiated. This is followed by rapid inflation and deflation of the stent-deployment valvuloplasty balloon, and termination of pacing and a return of a normal rhythm.
- Once the catheter is pulled back, the stent-valve will cover the native aortic leaflets and fit tightly in the aortic annulus. Angiography of the right and left coronary arteries is performed to assess blood flow. The femoral artery is repaired, and the sheath is removed.

Pathophysiology

Aortic stenosis. See under cardiac valve replacement.

Management

- Postoperative care: Monitor vital signs and intake and output.
- Monitor central venous pressures.
- Check femoral sites, dressings for drainage, hematoma, erythema.
- Assess bilateral lower extremities for warmth, color, sensation, and movement every 15 min for first hour, then hourly × 4 hr (or per hospital protocol).
- Keep affected limb straight for 8 hr.
- Head of bed should be elevated **no** more than 30°.
- Maintain bedrest for 12–24 hr post procedure; then the patient must ambulate.
- Assess neurological status frequently.
- Medicate for pain as needed.
- Administer IV fluids as ordered for 24 hr post-op.
- Monitor CBC and BMP labs.
- Provide continuous ECG monitoring.
- Administer clopidogrel (Plavix).

Endoscopic (Minimally Invasive) Coronary Artery Bypass Graft

- This less invasive cardiac surgical technique employs smaller incisions and totally "robotic" surgery using a computer-enhanced telemanipulation system. Saphenous vein harvesting can also be accomplished through small incisions using video-based surgical techniques, decreasing the morbidity associated with leg incision (pain, infection) and permitting more rapid recovery.

- **The term minimally invasive CABG** is applied to procedures that use alternatives to standard median sternotomy and off-pump CABG or on-pump CABG when a sternotomy is utilized. Two alternative techniques are used: beating heart CABG surgery and MID CABG off pump.
- **Less invasive minimal access CABG surgeries** emphasize the use of a limited thoracotomy incision as an alternative to a sternotomy, with either direct thoracoscopic or robotic-assisted left and right internal mammary artery harvesting and direct LIMA to coronary artery anastomotic techniques for myocardial stabilization.
- **Beating heart CABG surgery** is performed with specialized platforms that enable myocardial surface stabilization and limit myocardial motion and by use of temporary endovascular shunts to limit ischemia.
- **MID CABG off pump:** The pericardium is opened, and cardiac motion is limited by the creation of accurate technical anastomosis and designed to minimize disruption of the adjacent beating heart. Cardiac motion can further be limited by use of pharmacological interventions that temporarily decrease the heart rate or cause transient cardiac astystole for several seconds. Refer to CABG surgery for the detailed description of the actual bypass procedure.

Management

Post-op care is generally the same as traditional CABG surgery.

Cardiac and Cardiopulmonary Transplant

Cardiac transplant is a surgical procedure to remove a diseased heart and replace it with a healthy donor heart. The same is true for lung transplant. Frequently both are done together for end-stage disease of the heart and lungs when no other therapies are viable.

End-stage heart disease includes congenital heart disease (single ventricle physiology, coronary sinusoids), cardiomyopathy (primary: idiopathic, familial, secondary pregnancy, drug-induced), and acquired heart disease (valvular disease).

Candidates for Heart Transplant

- HF
- CAD with intractable angina symptoms
- Cardiomyopathy
- Pulmonary hypertension with irreversible right heart failure
- Sarcoidosis of the heart and lungs
- Ventricular dysrhythmias unresponsive to medical or surgery therapy
- Primary cardiac tumors with no evidence of spread to other body systems

Candidates for Lung Transplant

- COPD (chronic obstructive pulmonary disease)
- Cystic fibrosis
- Idiopathic pulmonary fibrosis
- Interstitial lung diseases
- Primary pulmonary hypertension

Diagnostic Tests Prior to Transplantation

A battery of tests are done prior to transplantation. These may include but are not limited to the following:

- Echocardiogram
- Right heart catheterization
- Pulmonary function tests
- Exercise treadmill test
- Abdominal ultrasound
- Chest x-rays
- CT
- Coronary angiogram
- Cardiac biopsy
- Chromosome testing
- Updating of immunizations
- Low PSA and negative Pap smear
- Lab tests: serum chemistries, CBC, human leukocyte antigen (HLA) antibody screening, viral antibody screening (HIV, cytomegalovirus, herpes virus, varicella, Epstein-Barr), platelet count, urinalysis
- Psychosocial history obtained

Postoperative Care

- Admit to cardiothoracic ICU; 24–48 hr on ventilator until anesthesia cleared from system.
- Insert Foley catheter to gravity, monitor output closely.
- Obtain daily chest x-ray.
- Monitor chest tube sites and drainage (generally 2–3 chest tubes in place).
- Perform pulmonary toilet measures hourly, once extubated.
- Perform and document complete nursing assessments frequently during first 12–24 hr after surgery.
- Watch for signs and symptoms of bleeding.
- Treat dysrhythmias.
- Prevent right-sided heart failure.
- Watch for early signs of rejection, infection, immunosuppressive issues.
- Monitor for signs of drug toxicity.
- Provide ICU care for about 3–5 days post-op.

- Prevent rejection: cyclosporine (Neoral), azathioprine (Imuran), prednisone, methylprednisolone (Solu-Cortef), tacrolimus (Prograf), mycophenolate mofetil (CellCept), sirolimus (Rapamycin, Rapamune), monoclonal antibodies or polyclonal antibodies.
- Highest risk for infection: 1 wk postop.

Signs and Symptoms of Rejection

Hyperacute rejection can occur immediately after transplantation in the OR. Acute rejection occurs within the first 3 mo after transplantation. Chronic rejection can occur any time after 3 mo of transplant.

- Low-grade fever with elevated WBC
- Fatigue
- SOB
- Pulmonary crackles with/without pulmonary edema
- Pericardial friction rub
- Arrhythmias, especially atrial flutter or fibrillation
- Decreased ECG voltage
- Increased JVD
- Signs of decreased cardiac output including hypotension with tachycardia
- Cardiac enlargement on x-ray
- Vascular degeneration
- Palpitations
- Nausea and vomiting

Other Complications

- Infection
- CAD
- GI complications related to medications

Infections of the Heart

Infective Endocarditis

Infective endocarditis is the inflammation of the innermost layer of the heart. It can include the heart valves, chordae tendineae, cardiac septum, or lining of the chambers. It is caused typically by bacterial infections (*Streptococcus viridans* or *Staphylococcus aureus*).

Pathophysiology

Microbe invades the valve leaflets → infection occurs, causing valve leaflets to be deformed.

Clinical Presentation

Endocarditis manifests as:

- Low-grade and intermittent fever
- Chills, night sweats
- Anorexia, weight loss
- Myalgia, arthralgia
- Extreme fatigue and malaise
- Nausea and vomiting
- Headache
- SOB
- Chest pain
- Abdominal pain
- Confusion, delirium
- Pain in the muscles, joints, and back
- Influenza-like symptoms
- Loud regurgitant murmur; pericardial rub or friction rub
- Possible embolic stroke with focal neurological deficits

Be suspicious if petechiae appear on the conjunctiva, neck, anterior chest, abdomen, or oral mucosa. Look for Janeway lesions (nontender macule) on patient's palms and soles, Osler's nodes (tender, erythematous, raised nodules) on fingers and toe pads, and splinter hemorrhages under fingernails. Roth's spots are white spots that can be seen on the retina.

Diagnostic Tests

- Transthoracic echocardiogram
- ECG
- Chest x-ray
- Abdominal CT or MRI
- Positive blood cultures
- Refer to the Duke Criteria for Infective Endocarditis found at: http://www. medcalc.com/endocarditis.html

Management

- Administer antimicrobial therapy.
- Priorities include supporting cardiac function, eradicating the infection, and preventing complications, such as systemic embolization and heart failure.
- Do not give anticoagulants because of risk of intracerebral hemorrhage.

Pericarditis

Pericarditis is inflammation of pericardium that can cause fluid to accumulate in the pericardial space resulting from idiopathic causes, infection (viral, bacterial, or fungal), MI, autoimmune reactions, certain drugs, cancer therapies, or trauma. Dressler's syndrome is a type of pericarditis following damage to heart tissue or the pericardium, such as a heart attack, surgery, or traumatic injury.

Pathophysiology

Primary illness of medical or surgical disorder can be the etiology → pericardium becomes inflamed → can lead to excess fluid accumulation or increased pressure on the heart leading to tamponade.

Clinical Presentation

Sharp, constant chest pain that is located in the midchest (retrosternal) is the most common symptom. A hallmark sign of pericarditis is if the patient leans forward while sitting to relieve chest pain. Pain may radiate to the neck, shoulders, and back; radiation to the ridge of the left trapezius muscle is specific for pericarditis. ECG changes are new widespread ST elevation or PR depression, and pericardial effusion may be present.

Depending on the cause, patient may also have fever, malaise, tachypnea, dyspnea, JVD, and tachycardia. Pericardial friction rub, heard in the lower sternal border, is the most important physical sign.

Diagnostic Tests

- ECG
- Echocardiogram
- Chest x-ray
- Lab work: cardiac markers, erythrocyte sedimentation rate (ESR), serum C-reactive protein
- Serum electrolytes, BUN, creatinine
- Complete blood count
- Urinalysis
- Blood cultures
- Additional lab work may include tuberculin skin test, antinuclear antibody titer (ANA), and/or HIV serology
- Transesophageal echocardiogram (TEE)

Management

- NSAIDs (ibuprofen or ASA or indomethacin) may be used for up to 2 wk except in acute MI or pericarditis.
- Add colchicine (Colcrys) for recurrent symptoms or continued symptoms >14 days.

- Monitor for cardiac tamponade.
- More severe pain can be controlled with morphine.
- If cause is infectious, antibiotics or antifungal drugs may be administered.
- Treatment consists of antibiotics specific to the pathogen for at least 6 wk.
- If a pericardiectomy is performed, continue assessments of VS, lab work, and the appearance of wounds and insertion sites of invasive lines.
- Other surgical procedures include pericardiocentesis, pericardial window, pericardiotomy.
- Monitor temperature and cardiac rhythm; assess for heart murmurs.
- Perform neurological assessments, inspect skin surfaces, and monitor drug peaks and troughs and urine output.
- Disease may progress to cardiac tamponade and chronic constrictive pericarditis.

Pacemakers/AICD

Pacemakers generate an electrical impulse that stimulates the myocardium to depolarize, thereby initiating a cardiac contraction. Aim is to keep the ventricles beating to sustain adequate BP to perfuse all organs sufficiently. Consists of a pulse generator and 1–3 leads with electrodes.

Pacemakers can also stimulate only selected areas of the heart. Codes have been established for general widespread use.

Position	I	II	III	IV	V
Category	Chamber(s) paced	Chamber(s) sensed	Response to sending	Rate modulation	Multisite pacing
	O = none A = atrium V = ventricle D = dual (A+V)	O = none A = atrium V = ventricle D = dual (A+V)	O = none T = triggered I = inhibited D = dual (T+I)	O = none R = rate modulation	O = none A = atrium V = ventricle D = dual (A+V)
Manufacturers' designation only	S = single (A or V)	S = single (A or V)			

- VVI mode: The ventricle is paced, sensed, and inhibited. The pacemaker fires if no QRS complex is sensed. The patient's rate is greater than the programmed rate and inhibits the pacemaker from firing. Most popular mode.
- DVI or AV sequential mode: The atrium is paced at the programmed rate → no ventricular activity during a certain interval → ventricle is paced.
- DDD or fully automated mode: Senses and paces both the atrium and ventricle and can inhibit either the atrium or ventricle if a patient's native or intrinsic beat is sensed.
- Position I: Heart chamber paced.
- Position II: Heart chamber where intrinsic electrical activity sensed.
- Position II: Pacemaker response to what it senses.
- Position IV: Presence (R) or absence (O) of rate modulation or rate responsiveness. Presence means that the pacemaker will alter its pacing rate to meet metabolic demands.
- Position V: Multisite pacing settings indicate the ability to stimulate more than 1 site in a chamber.
- Fixed rate pacemakers (asynchronous) discharge at a preset rate (usually 70–80 bpm) regardless of the patient's own electrical activity.
- Demand (synchronous) pacemakers discharge only when the patient's HR < the pacemaker's preset rate.
- Pacemakers may also be classified as temporary or permanent. Temporary pacemakers are used in emergency situations and may serve as a bridge to a permanent pacemaker. The pulse generator is located externally. The pulse generator is implanted internally in permanent pacemakers.
- Temporary pacemakers include transvenous, epicardial, transcutaneous, and transthoracic.
- Transvenous pacing: A lead wire is passed through the brachial, internal or external jugular, subclavian, or femoral vein to the myocardium.
- Epicardial pacing is used with cardiac surgical patients. Epicardial wires are attached to the epicardium during surgery.
- Transthoracic pacing is used as a last resort, with limited success rates. A pacing needle is inserted directly into the anterior wall of the heart.

Transcutaneous Pacemakers

Transcutaneous pacemakers are used for noninvasive temporary pacing using two large external electrodes. The electrodes are attached to an external pulse generator, which operates on alternating current or battery. The generator emits electrical pulses, which are transmitted through the electrodes and then transcutaneously to stimulate ventricular depolarization when the patient's heart rate is slower than the rate set on the pacemaker. Used as an emergency measure, a transcutaneous pacemaker should be used for 48–72 hr only. Electrodes should be changed every 24 hr minimally.

Permanent Pacemakers

Permanent pacing is performed for the resolution of nontemporary conduction disorders, including complete heart block and sick sinus syndrome. Permanent pacemakers are usually powered by a lithium battery and have an average life span of 10 yr.

Indications

- Class I: The procedure should be performed.
- Class IIa: It is reasonable to perform the procedure, but additional studies with focused objectives are needed.
- Class IIb: The procedure may be considered, but additional studies with broad objectives are needed.
- Class III: The procedure should not be performed; it is not helpful and may be harmful.

In 2008 the American College of Cardiology (ACC), the American Heart Association (AHA), and the Heart Rhythm Society (HRS) jointly published guidelines for pacemaker insertion indications, which was updated in 2012:

- Class I indications
  - Sinus node dysfunction
  - Acquired atrioventricular block in adults
  - Chronic bifascicular block
  - After acute MI
  - Hypersensitive carotid sinus syndrome and neurocardiogenic syncope
  - After cardiac transplantation
  - Pacing to prevent tachycardia
  - Congenital heart disease
- Class IIa indications
  - Sinus node dysfunction
  - Acquired atrioventricular block
  - Hypersensitive carotid sinus syndrome and neurocardiogenic syncope
  - Congenital heart disease
  - Pacing to prevent tachycardia
  - Permanent pacemakers that automatically detect and pace to terminate tachycardia
- Class IIb indications
  - Sinus node dysfunction
  - Acquired atrioventricular block in adults
  - Chronic bifascicular block
  - After acute MI
  - Hypersensitive carotid sinus syndrome and neurocardiogenic syncope
  - After cardiac transplant

- Pacing to prevent tachycardia
- Congenital heart disease

Contraindications

- Local infection at implantation site
- Active systemic infection with bacteremia
- Severe bleeding tendencies (relative contraindication)
- Active anticoagulation therapy (relative contraindication)
- Severe lung disease and positive end-expiratory pressure ventilation (relative contraindication for internal jugular and subclavian access.

Procedure

- Performed in an electrophysiology (EP) lab or in a cardiac catheterization lab. Usually done using local anesthesia.
- Small incision is made at the insertion site (usually right or left subclavian); a sheath or introducer is inserted into the subclavian vein; a lead wire is threaded through the introducer into the vessel; and the lead wire is then advanced into the atrium, ventricle, or both (depending on the type of pacemaker).
- Once the lead wire is in the proper position, it is tested to verify proper location and to make sure it is functioning properly. The number of leads placed (1, 2, or 3) depends on the type of pacemaker.
- Once the lead wires are tested, an incision is made under the clavicle. The pacemaker generator is slipped under the skin through the incision after the lead wire is attached to the generator. An ECG is obtained to verify the pacer is working correctly.
- The incision is then closed with sutures, adhesive strips, or surgical glue; a dry sterile dressing is then applied.

Postoperative Care

Patients are not always admitted or returned to the ICU post procedure; a telemetry floor may be appropriate.

- Continuous cardiac monitoring. A pacemaker-generated impulse should appear as a spike on the ECG. The spike indicates the pacemaker has fired. Pacemaker rhythm:
  - Rate: Varies according to the preset pacemaker rate and patient's native heart rate.
  - Rhythm: Irregular for demand pacemaker unless patient is 100% based with no native beats.
  - P wave: None for ventricular pacemaker. P waves may be seen but unrelated to QRS. Atrial or dual chambered pacemakers should have P wave after each atrial spike.
  - PR interval: None for ventricular pacing. Atrial or dual chambered pacing should produce constant PR intervals.
  - QRS: Wide (>0.10 sec.) after each ventricular spike in a paced beat. Patient's native QRS will look different from paced QRS. Atrial pacing only, QRS may be normal.

■ Obtain a 12-lead ECG.
■ Assess VS per hospital protocol. Assess peripheral pulses.
■ Assess LOC.
■ Administer antibiotics (cefazolin, vancomycin).
■ Assess dressing for bleeding, drainage, or signs of infection.
■ If epicardial wires present, clean site and cover wires per hospital policy.
■ Monitor CBC, BMP.
■ Administer oral pain medication as needed.
■ Patients with pacemakers may be defibrillated. Avoid placing the defib-
   rillator paddles or pads closer than 5 inches from the pacemaker battery
   pack or pulse generator.
■ Patient education is crucial: activity level, signs of pacemaker malfunction,
   signs of infection, electrical safety precautions, medication usage. Provide
   patient with identification card related to pacemaker. Consider telemonitor-
   ing of these patients for compliance, pacemaker function, and avoidance of
   complications.

Complications

■ Pacemaker malfunction:
   ○ Failure to discharge: Pacemaker fails to fire. Seen as patient's HR
   ○ Failure to capture: Pacing stimulus not followed by depolarization of
      programmed rate
   ○ Oversensing: Pacemaker detects noncardiac electrical events (electro-
      atrium and/or ventricle
   ○ Undersensing: Pacemaker cannot sense patient's intrinsic beats, with
      magnetic interference, large T waves) as depolarization
      resulting inappropriately placed pacemaker artifacts
■ Pneumothorax
■ Ventricular irritability
■ Perforation of ventricular wall or septum
■ Catheter or lead dislodgment
■ Infection
■ Hematoma
■ Abdominal twitching or hiccups
■ Pocket erosion

Automatic Implantable Cardioverter-Defibrillator Device (AICD)

■ The AICD continuously monitors the patient's heart rhythm, diagnoses any
   rhythm changes, and treats life-threatening ventricular arrhythmias.
■ Main indications for use of an AICD relate to secondary prevention in
   patients with prior sustained ventricular tachycardia (VT), ventricular
   fibrillation (VF), or resuscitated sudden cardiac death (SCD) thought to

be caused by VT/VF as well as primary prevention in patients at risk of life-threatening VT/VF.

■ The American Heart Association (AHA), American College of Cardiology (ACC), and the Heart Rhythm Society (HRS) updated guidelines for managing patients with ventricular arrhythmias and the prevention of sudden cardiac death in 2017.

Indications for ICD Therapy

Secondary prevention: Implantation of an ICD is recommended for the secondary prevention of death resulting from VT/VF in the following settings:

■ Patients with prior episode of resuscitated VT/VF or sustained hemodynamically unstable VT in whom a completely reversible cause cannot be identified. This includes patients with a variety of underlying heart diseases and those with idiopathic VT/VF and congenital long QT syndrome, but **not** patients who have VT/VF limited to the first 48 hr after an AMI.

■ Patients with episodes of spontaneous sustained VT in the presence of heart disease (valvular, ischemic, hypertrophic, dilated, or infiltrative cardiomyopathies) and other settings (i.e., channelopathies).

Primary prevention: Implantation of an ICD is recommended for the primary prevention of life-threatening VT/VF in patients at risk of SCD from VT/VF who have optimal medical management (including use of beta blockers and ACE-IS), including:

■ Patients with prior myocardial infarction (at least 40 days ago) and left ventricular ejection fraction ≤30%.

■ Patients with cardiomyopathy, New York Heart Association functional class II or III, and left ventricular ejection fraction <35%. Patients with nonischemic cardiomyopathy generally require optimal medical therapy for 3 mo with documentation of persistent left ventricular ejection fraction <35% at that time. Recommended patients be evaluated at least 3 mo after revascularization (CABG or stent placement).

Procedure

Refer to pacemaker insertion.

Management

Post-op care: Refer to Pacemakers.

Cardiac Tamponade

Cardiac tamponade is the acute compression of the heart caused by excessive fluid or blood in the pericardial space. This results in accumulated pressure in the pericardial sac and affects the heart's function, especially cardiac output. Normal pericardial fluid volume = 10–30 mL, but a rapid accumulation of 50–100 ml of fluid can be fatal. It is a medical emergency that can result in pulmonary edema, shock, and death.

Pathophysiology

Causes: accidents, stab wounds, gunshot wounds, rupture of tumors, obstruction of lymphatic or venous flow, pericardial effusion → accumulate blood in the pericardial sac → ↑ venous pressure → compress all four chambers of the heart → RA and RV are compressed → ↑ RA filling during diastole → ↑ venous blood returns to RA → ↑ venous pressure → JVD, edema, hepatomegaly, ↑ DBP → continued compression of the heart → ↓ diastolic filling of ventricles → ↓ SV, ↓ CO, ↓ tissue perfusion → body attempts to increase blood volume, increase SV ↑ → workload of the heart → tachycardia → all these complications last for a limited amount of time → shock, cardiac arrest, or death if not immediately corrected.

Clinical Manifestations

First Signs
- Anxiety and restlessness, syncope
- SOB, dyspnea on exertion, orthopnea, cough
- Unwillingness to lie flat
- Cool, diaphoretic skin
- Sense of impending doom

Classic Signs
- Beck's triad: muffled heart sounds, increased JVD, and hypotension
- Narrow pulse pressure (↓ SBP and ↓ DBP)
- Hemodynamics: ↑ CVP >20 mm Hg, ↓ PCWP, ↓ CO
- Tachycardia
- Weak, thready pulse

Late Signs
- Pulsus paradoxus (↓ SBP of more than 10 mm Hg on inspiration)
- Electrical alternans (alternating levels of voltage in P waves and QRS complexes in all leads and possibly in T waves)

Diagnostic Tests
- Chest x-ray
- Echocardiogram
- ECG
- CT, MRI

82

Management

- If acute onset, call MD stat, obtain stat 2-D echocardiogram and stat chest x-ray.
- Obtain stat lab work.
- MD will place pulmonary artery catheter.
- Place patient in supine position with HOB elevated 30°–60°.
- Assess O_2 saturation levels and administer O_2 by cannula, mask or intubate.
- If on mechanical ventilation, no positive pressure used.
- Give sedatives; administer morphine for chest pain.
- Monitor cardiovascular, respiratory, neurological, and renal function status.
- Assess hemodynamics.
- Obtain 12-lead ECG, and provide continuous ECG monitoring. Notify MD of increasing dyspnea and new-onset arrhythmias.
- Administer inotropic drugs (dobutamine) for low BP.
- Consider volume expansion with blood, plasma, dextran, or isotonic sodium chloride solution, as necessary, to maintain adequate intravascular volume.
- Prepare patient for surgery or procedure to remove pericardial fluid: pericardiotomy, pericardiocentesis, surgical creation of pericardial window. Other procedures may be considered for recurrent cardiac tamponade or pericardial effusion. Removal of as little as 10–20 mL of fluid may relieve symptoms.

ACLS Algorithms: Cardiac/Respiratory Arrest

Based on the Adult Basic Life Support: American Heart Association Guidelines for Cardiopulmonary Resuscitation and Emergency Cardiovascular Care with 2017 Focused Updates. Refer to: http://circ.ahajournals.org/content/122/18_suppl_3/S685 .full.pdf+html for full report.

Ventricular Fibrillation (VF) or Pulseless Ventricular Tachycardia (VT)

- **Shock:** Biphasic: 120 J; monophasic: 200 J. Reassess rhythm.
- **CPR:** Immediately perform 5 cycles of CPR (should last about 2 min).
- **Epinephrine:** 1 mg IV or IO (2–2.5 mg, endotracheal tube) every 3–5 min *or* **vasopressin:** 40 units IV or IO, one time only. May use to replace 1st or 2nd dose of epinephrine (given without interrupting CPR).
- **Shock:** Biphasic: 150 J then 200 J; monophasic: 300 J then 360 J. Reassess rhythm.

- **Consider antiarrhythmics** (given without interrupting CPR):
  - **Amiodarone:** 300 mg IV or IO, may repeat 150 mg in 3–5 min.
  - **Lidocaine:** 1.0–1.5 mg/kg IV or IO, may repeat 0.5–0.75 mg/kg q5–10 min. max 3 mg/kg.
  - **Magnesium:** 1–2 g IV or IO for torsades de pointes.
- A 2011 study published in *Circulation* showed that patients with a shockable rhythm (VF or pulseless VT) had better survival rates if CPR is paused for only 10 sec or less before delivery of electric shock to the heart (preshock pause) or a total of 20 sec or less pause in chest compressions both before and after defibrillatory shock (perishock pause).
- 76% of patients show signs of ongoing instability for several hours prior to cardiac arrest.
- 70% of patients show signs of respiratory distress within 8 hr of arrest.
- 66% of patients show abnormal signs and symptoms within 6 hr of arrest.

Asystole or Pulseless Electrical Activity (PEA)

- Resume CPR for 5 cycles (should last about 2 min).
- **Epinephrine:** 1 mg IV or IO (2 to 2.5 mg ET) every 3–5 min *or* **vasopressin:** 40 units IV or IO, one time only. May use to replace 1st or 2nd dose of epinephrine (given without interrupting CPR).

Intra-aortic Balloon Pump Counterpulsation (IABP)

IABP counterpulsation provides temporary mechanical circulatory support. Goals of IABP counterpulsation: increase O_2 to myocardium and coronary arteries, decrease LV workload by decreasing impedance to ejection (afterload), and increase cardiac output. An IABP device consists of a 30-cm polyurethane balloon attached to one end of a large-bore catheter. The device is inserted into the femoral artery at the groin, either percutaneously or via arteriotomy, with the balloon wrapped tightly around the catheter. Once inserted, the catheter is advanced up the aorta until the tip lies just beyond the origin of the left subclavian artery. When in place, the balloon wrapping is released to allow periodic balloon inflations.

Effects

The intra-aortic balloon is inflated with helium at the onset of each diastolic period (middle of T wave), when the aortic valve closes. The balloon is deflated at the onset of ventricular systole, just before aortic valve opens (prior to QRS complex). An arterial waveform can be used as an alternative to ECG triggering. Inflation of the balloon increases the peak diastolic pressure and displaces blood toward the periphery. Deflation of the balloon decreases the end-diastolic pressure, which reduces impedance to flow when aortic valve opens at onset of systole. This decreases ventricular afterload and promotes stroke volume, thus increasing coronary artery perfusion and blood flow during diastole.

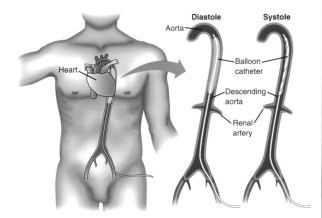

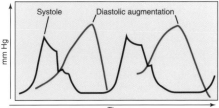

IABP Waveforms

Indications

- Complement to cardiopulmonary bypass and low cardiac output after cardiac surgery
- Bridge to VAD, CABG, or cardiac transplant
- AMI with cardiogenic shock
- Decompensated heart failure
- Acute mitral valve insufficiency or regurgitation
- Ventricular septal defect or papillary muscle ruptures
- Severe unstable or intractable angina
- Septic shock

Timing

- Balloon should inflate at or slightly above the dicrotic notch.
- A crisp V shape should appear on inflation.
- Diastolic augmentation peak > preceding systolic peak.
- The following systolic peak (assisted systole) < preceding systole (unassisted systole).
- The IABP should be set on a 1:2 augmentation to assess timing and then 1:1 or 1:3 augmentation after timing has been optimized.
- Avoid early or late inflation and deflation.

Management

- Routine critical care nursing practices are followed.
- Instruct patient not to sit up, bend knee, or flex hip >45°. Keep HOB <45°.
- Provide continuous ECG monitoring.
- Arterial line and pulmonary artery catheter are in place.
- Assess insertion site for bleeding and infection.

Complications

- Balloon leakage, rupture, or entrapment. The catheter can migrate and occlude subclavian artery.
- Lower limb ischemia and compartment syndrome of cannulated extremity.
- Arterial occlusion → mesenteric infarction.
- Catheter-associated infection.

Contraindications

- Aortic insufficiency and regurgitation
- Aortic aneurysm and dissection
- Recently placed (within 12 mo) prosthetic graft in thoracic aorta

Induced or Therapeutic Hypothermia

Also called targeted temperature management. To reduce the damage to brain cells through reduction of the brain's metabolic activity, hypothermia is intentionally induced by bringing the core body temperature down to 32°C–34°C (89.6°F–93.2°F). It is recommended that therapeutic hypothermia be used for up to 24 hr, although little evidence supports this time frame. Cerebral metabolism ↓ 6%–10% for every 1° decrease in body temperature. As cerebral metabolism ↓ → brain O_2 requirements ↓. Goals: ↓ ICP, ↓ HR, ↓ brain's O_2 demand to obtain good neurological outcome. Indications for medically induced hypothermia include:

- Ischemic cerebral or spinal injury, including stroke recovery
- Cerebral edema and increased intracranial pressure
- Heart surgery
- Patients with asystole, pulseless electrical activity, or cardiac arrest resulting from ventricular fibrillation (VF) or ventricular tachycardia (VT); this is most effective within 1 hr of cardiac arrest and no later than 10 hr after return of spontaneous circulation

The three phases in instituting induced hypothermia are induction, maintenance, and rewarming.

Hypothermia may be accomplished by several methods:

- Rapid infusion of ice-cold IV fluids; use 0.9% NS or LR at 30 mL/kg
- NG lavage with ice water
- Evaporative cooling of the external body surface
- External cooling with ice packs (axilla, groin, around head) or special cooling blankets, iced wet sheets, fans, gel pads
- Invasive cooling catheters

The patient may be rewarmed through the use of:

- Cardiopulmonary bypass
- Warm IV fluid administration
- Warm humidified O_2 administration via ventilator
- Warm peritoneal lavage
- Warming blankets and over-the-bed heaters

Caution should be taken with active core rewarming because VF can occur as the patient's temperature increases.

- Monitor for hypotension
- Rewarm slowly at 0.3°C–0.5°C/hr
- If no signs of neurological improvement 72 hr after rewarming and discontinuation of neuromuscular blockers, determine brain death and seek full neurological evaluation

Management

- Monitor BP. Arterial line is preferred.
- Provide continuous ECG monitoring and monitor for sinus bradycardia, prolonged PR interval, widened QRS, prolonged QT interval, atrial fibrillation, VT, and VF. Avoid atropine.
- Consider pacemaker or AICD.
- Monitor hemodynamics. Pulmonary artery catheter is preferred. IABP may be indicated.
- Administer vasopressors as needed.
- Monitor for seizures.
- Monitor fluids and electrolytes, especially K⁺ and glucose levels. Induction causes mild diuresis. Provide fluid replacement. Hyperglycemia can occur during maintenance phase, and hypoglycemia can occur during rewarming.
- Consider CRRT.
- Prevent skin breakdown resulting from vasoconstriction from cold. Consider prone position.
- Ileus is common during hypothermia.
- Hypothermia suppresses inflammatory response ← infection. Hand hygiene and infection control practices are imperative.
- Assess for bleeding. For every 1°C drop in temperature, coagulation-factor function ↑ by 10% and affects the coagulation cascade.
- Obtain oral or axillary temperatures only or use temperature probe, esophageal bladder, pulmonary artery catheter, or other methods.
- Prevent shivering through the use of sedation and neuromuscular blockade. Administer chlorpromazine (Thorazine) or diazepam (Valium).
- Hypothermia ↓ body's ability to respond to stimulation, making assessment of sedation level difficult. Use bispectral index monitors or continuous EEG monitoring.
- Assessing level of neuromuscular blockade using train-of-four monitoring not always reliable. Refer to Tab 1, Basics.
- Hypothermia affects drug metabolism. Lower doses of drugs may be needed.
- Prepare patient for immediate coronary angiography and/or PCI.

ECGs

12-Lead ECG

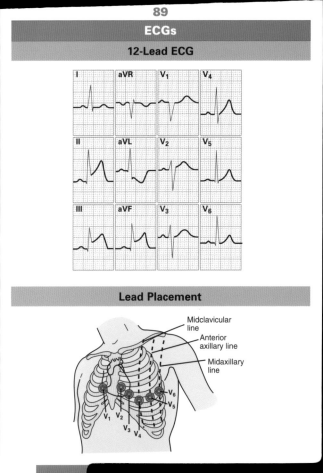

Lead Placement

ECG Changes Reflective of MI Locations

Location of MI	ECG Changes	Coronary Artery Involvement
Anterior	ST elevation, tall T waves, large R waves in V_3, V_4	LAD
	Reciprocal changes in II, III, aVF May progress to cardiogenic shock and AV heart block	
Inferior	ST elevation in II, III, aVF ST depression in I, aVL	RCA
Lateral	ST elevation in I, aVL, V_5, V_6 May see reciprocal changes in V1-V3	Circumflex
Posterior	Because there are no leads that look directly at posterior wall, diagnosed by tall R waves and ST depression in V_1–V_4, 15-lead ECG helpful in diagnosis	RCA or Circumflex
Anteroseptal	No normal R waves in V_1–V_4 Pathological Q waves	LAD

Hemodynamics of Dysrhythmias

Atrial Dysrhythmias

Atrial dysrhythmias are caused by increased automaticity in the atria. The patient may complain of palpitations or "heart racing." Loss of atrial contraction → shortens diastole → loss of atrial kick (25%–30% of CO) → ↓ CO → ↓ coronary perfusion → ischemic myocardial changes. Atrial flutter or fibrillation can lead to a pulmonary embolus, stroke, or MI. These patients should be taking anticoagulants. Calculation for Atrial Fibrillation Stroke Risk found at: http://www .mdcalc.com/cha2ds2-vasc-score-for-atrial-fibrillation-stroke-risk/ Surgical ablation via a Cox-Maze procedure during mitral valve repair or replacement has been shown to be an effective treatment for atrial fibrillation.

Causes
- Amphetamines
- Cocaine
- Decongestants
- Hypokalemia
- Hyperthyroidism
- COPD

- Pericarditis
- Digoxin toxicity
- Hypothermia
- Alcohol intoxication
- Pulmonary edema

Ventricular Dysrhythmias

Ventricular dysrhythmias are caused by increased automaticity in the ventricles. PVCs can be manifested as complaints of "heart skipping a beat." This dysrhythmia can lead to bradycardia → ↓ CO → ↓ BP and eventually VT, VF, and death.

Bradycardia

Bradycardia is defined as a heart rate less than 60 bpm. ↓ HR → ↓ CO → ↓ BP → ↓ perfusion to brain, heart, kidneys, lung, and skin.

Causes
- Vomiting
- Gagging
- Valsalva maneuver
- ETT suctioning

Symptoms
- Chest pain
- SOB
- Altered mental status
- Signs of ↓ CO: dizziness, weakness, low BP

Treatment Considerations
- Atropine
- Epinephrine
- Isoproterenol (Isuprel)
- Pacemaker
- Dopamine if hypotensive

Tachycardia

Tachycardia is defined as a heart rate greater than 100 bpm. ↑ ↑ HR can compromise cardiac output (CO) by ↓ ventricular filling → ↓ SV → ↓ CO → ↑ workload of the heart → ↑ O_2 consumption.

Causes
- Bronchodilators
- Caffeine
- Nicotine

CV

- Pain
- Fever
- Pulmonary embolism
- Hypoxia
- Heart failure
- Stress
- Anxiety

Symptoms

- Altered LOC
- Chest pain or discomfort
- Palpitations
- SOB
- Diaphoresis
- Hypotension
- Jugular venous distention

Treatment Considerations

- Carotid massage
- Valsalva maneuver
- Cardiovert at 100–360 J
- Radiofrequency ablation
- Pacemaker
- If arrhythmia converts to pulseless VT or VF → defibrillate
- Implantable cardioverter defibrillator (ICD), if indicated

QTc Prolongation

- Acquired drug-induced cardiac conduction abnormality causing delayed repolarization of ventricular myocardium.
- Normal QT interval is <440 msec. QT intervals 440–460 msec are considered borderline for men and 440–470 msec for women. Greater values for each gender are considered a prolonged QT interval.
- QT interval shortens with tachycardia and lengthens with bradycardia. A rate corrected (QTc) is clinically calculated. No one best method to calculate. QTc interval >510 msec is clinically significant. Quick calculation method: preceding RR interval + 2. A calculator for corrected QT interval can be found at http://www.mdcalc.com/corrected-qt-interval-qtc/ or http://www.medical-calculator.nl/calculator/QTc/
- Criteria for QT monitoring (at least one must be met)
  - Use of a QT-prolonging medication
  - Presence of cardiac arrhythmias causing severe bradycardia or long pauses
  - Patients with hypomagnesemia or hypokalemia

Causes

- Select antimicrobials: macrolides, fluoroquinolones, azole antifungals
- Select antiarrhythmics: classes Ia, Ic, III
- Select antipsychotics: haloperidol, risperidone, and others
- Select antidepressants
- Select amphetamines and anticholinergics
- Select sympathomimetics and vasodilators
- Methadone and oxycodone
- Phenothiazines and protease inhibitors
- Benadryl and nonsedating antihistamines; select decongestants
- Select diuretics
- Select antiemetics: ondansetron (Zofran), cisapride, prochlorperazine, and metoclopramide (Reglan)
- Hypokalemia and hypomagnesemia
- Bradycardia, complete heart block, and long sinus pauses
- SAH and stroke
- HF

Complications of Prolonged QT

Torsades de pointes (TdP): a fatal ventricular arrhythmia causing syncope, palpitations, dizziness, seizures, VT, or no symptoms. ECG findings: QTc >0.50 msec, frequent polymorphic PVCs and couplets, T-wave alternans, prominent U waves (>1 mm) that may be fused with T wave, nonsustained polymorphic VT, rate 200–250 bpm, frequently preceded by a long RR interval followed by a short RR interval and a PVC, more organized than VF, duration may be short and may self-terminate.

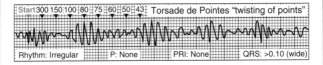

Start 300 150 100 80 75 60 50 43 — Torsade de Pointes "twisting of points"

| Rhythm: Irregular | P: None | PRI: None | QRS: >0.10 (wide) |

Management

- Print a long rhythm strip to determine the average QT interval.
- Obtain a 12-lead ECG with a lead of well-defined T waves. Use same lead for QTc monitoring.
- Administer bolus of 50% magnesium sulfate 2 g IV over 1–2 min followed by another such bolus if required; a continuous infusion of 2–4 mg/min regardless of serum magnesium level may be required in accordance with hospital policy.
- Administer beta blockers if QTc >460 ms in women or >440 ms in men.

- Perform overdrive transvenous cardiac pacing.
- Correct electrolyte abnormalities.
- Consider isoproterenol and atropine in resistant cases or prior to pacing.
- Review medication profile and discontinue offending drug.
- Perform defibrillation if prolonged. Consider implantable cardiac defibrillator.

Torsades de Pointes

- Rate >200
- Rhythm regular or irregular
- PR not applicable
- QRS >0.12/sec, wide and bizarre, oscillating character of QRS complexes (bigger-smaller-bigger, etc.)
- T wave opposite of QRS but may not be seen, embedded in QRS
- Causes: quinidine, amiodarone, sotalol, flecainide, or any antiarrhythmics that increase QT interval
  - Low K, low magnesium
  - Select antihistamines and antibiotics
- May result in cardiac arrest
- Treatment:
  - IV magnesium
  - Cardioversion
  - Defibrillation
  - O_2
  - AICD
  - Catheter ablation

Determining Rate and Measurement

To figure out rate (regular rhythms only), you can do one of the following:

Count the number of QRS complexes (regular rhythms only) in a 6-sec strip and multiply by 10.

Irregular rhythms should be counted for an entire minute.

Divide the number of large boxes between two R waves into 300.

Remember the number sequence below and find an R wave that falls on a heavy line. Starting from the next heavy line, count 300, 150, 100, and so forth, and whatever line the next R wave falls on is the heart rate (see below for example).

| 1st R wave | 300 | 150 | 100 | 75 | 60 | 50 | 43 |

Next R wave here would be 150 bpm.

Next R wave here would be 60 bpm.

Inherent rates of different cardiac regions:
SA Node....................60–100 bpm
AV Node....................40–60 bpm
Ventricles..................20–40 bpm

One **small** box represents 0.04 sec and is 1 mm².

One **big** box represents 0.20 sec and is 5 mm².

Normal Cardiac Cycle and Measurements

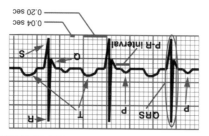

Normal Rate → **60 to 100 bpm**
Normal PR → 0.12–0.20 sec
Normal QRS → 0.08–0.12 sec
P wave ← atrial depolarization; **QRS** ← ventricular depolarization; **T wave** ← ventricular repolarization

Quick Guide to Analyzing the ECG

- Determine the overall rate: <60 bpm → bradycardia, >100 bpm → tachycardia.
- Determine the regularity: regular or irregular.
  - If irregular, is there any pattern?
- Examine the P waves.
  - Is there a P wave before each QRS? Is there more than 1 P wave?
  - Are P waves absent?
  - What is the configuration of the P wave? Round? Saw toothed?
  - Do they look the same?
  - Do any occur earlier or later than expected?
  - Are any P waves located within the QRS or T wave?
- Determine the PR interval.
  - Is it normal, prolonged, or shortened?
  - Can it be measured?
  - Is it the same for each beat? Any pattern?
- Examine the QRS complex.
  - Is there a QRS after each P wave?
  - Do they look the same?
  - Do any occur earlier than expected?
  - Is there a pattern to QRS complexes occurring early?

Normal Cardiac Rhythm Parameters

NSR	• 60–100 bpm
Bradycardia	• <60 bpm; consider sinus bradycardia, AV block
Tachycardia	• >100 bpm; consider atrial fibrillation, atrial flutter, supraventricular tachycardia, ventricular tachycardia
PR interval	• 0.12–0.20 sec
	• >0.20 sec; consider AV block
	• <0.12 sec; consider junctional rhythm
	• Unable to determine; consider atrial arrhythmia, junctional arrhythmia; examine QRS to determine whether ventricular arrhythmia
P wave	• Generally round
	• Saw toothed → consider atrial flutter
	• Spiked, nonrounded; consider atrial fibrillation or PACs
QRS	• 0.06–0.10 sec
	• Wide, bizarre; consider PVC, VT

If baseline is grossly irregular with no discernible P waves, consider VT. Flat baseline, asystole; begin CPR for either dysrhythmia.

ECK Interpretation

Rate: _____

Rhythm: _____

P waves: _____

PR Intervals: _____

ORS: _____

QT: _____

Interpretation _____

Supraventricular Tachycardia (SVT)

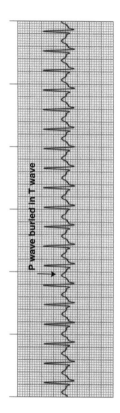

P wave buried in T wave

- **Rate:** 150–250 bpm
- **Rhythm:** Usually regular
- **PR interval:** Unable to determine
- **P waves:** Usually hidden in preceding T wave
- **QRS:** 0.06–0.10 sec, >0.10 sec if conducted through the ventricles
- **Causes:** Nicotine, stress, anxiety, caffeine
- **Management:** Vagal maneuver, adenosine (Adenocard, Adenoscan), amiodarone (Cordarone, Pacerone), diltiazem (Cardizem), propafenone (Rythmol), flecainide (Tambocor); cardioversion or overdrive pacing if drugs ineffective

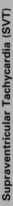

Atrial Flutter

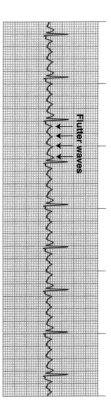

Flutter waves

AV node conducts impulses to the ventricle with varying degrees of block (2:1 →2 flutter waves:1 QRS; 4:1 → 4 flutter waves: 1 QRS); loss of atrial kick. Seen in coronary artery disease and valvular disease.

■ ■ ■ ■ ■ **Atrial rate:** 250–400 bpm
■ ■ ■ ■ **PR interval:** Unable to determine
■ ■ ■ **Rhythm:** Regular or irregular depending if combination of degrees of block (e.g., 2:1 + 4:1)
■ ■ **P waves:** Saw-toothed flutter waves
■ **Ventricular rate:** Slow or fast depending on degree of block
QRS: Normal or narrow
Management: Diltiazem; propafenone (rhythmol), flecainide (tambocor), acebutolol, esmolol, metoprolol, atenolol, pindolol, digoxin, amiodarone, electrical cardioversion if ventricular rate >150 bpm, radiofrequency ablation; anticoagulate. Consider Tikosyn (dofetilide) if refractory to cardioversion. Assess for and treat OSA

Atrial Fibrillation

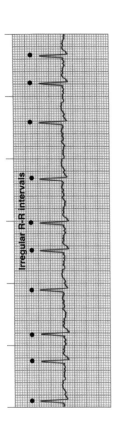

Irregular R-R intervals

Atrium quivers instead of contracting; loss of atrial kick. Mural thrombi can lead to pulmonary embolism or stroke. Symptoms include palpitations, fatigue, malaise, pulse deficit ↑ risk of myocardial ischemia.

- **Atrial rate:** 400–600 bpm
- **PR interval:** Unable to determine
- **Rhythm:** Irregularly irregular
- **P waves:** None; fibrillatory waves
- **Ventricular rate:** Normal or fast
- **QRS:** Usually narrow
- **Management:** Same as atrial flutter; ibutilide (Corvert) after cardioversion; anticoagulate. Consider Tikosyn (dofetilide) if refractory to cardioversion. Assess for and treat OSA. Consider Cox-Maze procedure during mitral valve repair or replacement

A3

Premature Ventricular Contraction (PVC)

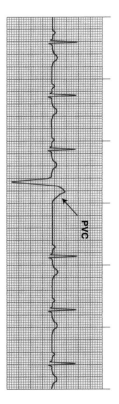

PVC

May be uniform (one ectopic focus or unifocal) or different foci (multifocal). Patient may complain of light-headedness, palpitations, heart skipping a beat.

- **P wave:** Absent before PVC
- **Rhythm:** Irregular where PVC occurs
- **QRS:** Wide, bizarre, >0.10 sec; may be followed by compensatory pause
- **Causes:** Healthy persons, caffeine, nicotine, stress, cardiac ischemia or infarction, digoxin toxicity, electrolyte imbalances, hypovolemia, fever, hypokalemia, hypoxia, hypermagnesemia, acid-base imbalance
- **Management:** Correct the cause; amiodarone, lidocaine

Ventricular Tachycardia (VT)

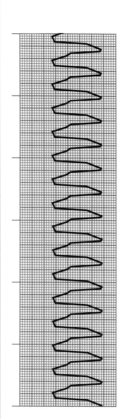

Three or more PVCs together with the same shape and amplitude.
Unstable rhythm. Easily progresses to VF if VT sustained and untreated. Patient may or may not have a pulse, no BP.

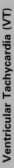

Atrial rate: Unable to determine; no P waves; no PR interval
Ventricular rate: 100–250 bpm
Rhythm: Usually regular
QRS: Wide & bizarre, >0.10 sec
Management: Epinephrine or vasopressin, amiodarone, procainamide, lidocaine, sotalol, immediate synchronized cardioversion; pulseless VT is treated the same as VF. Consider AICD

Ventricular Fibrillation (VF)

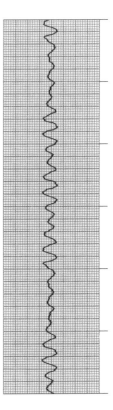

Chaotic pattern. No effective ventricular contraction. No CO, no pulse, no BP. Brain death occurs within 4-6 min if untreated.

- **Atrial rate:** Unable to determine; no P waves; no PR interval
- **Ventricular rate:** Fibrillatory waves with no pattern
- **Rhythm:** Irregular
- **Management:** Amiodarone, procainamide, lidocaine, magnesium sulfate, immediate defibrillation at 200–360 J; CPR with epinephrine, vasopressin, and sodium bicarbonate; intubate, IV access if none present, induce mild hypothermia 32°C–34°C (89.6°F–93.2°F). Consider AICD

Torsades de Pointes (TdP)

Refer to page 93, Complications of Prolonged QT.

First-Degree AV Block

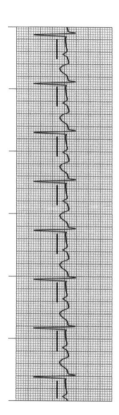

Problem in the conduction system. May progress to more severe block. Patient usually has no symptoms and no hemodynamic changes.

- **P wave:** Present, before each QRS
- **Rhythm:** Regular
- **PR interval:** >0.20 sec
- **QRS:** Normal
- **Management:** Correct the cause, monitor closely; usually benign. Evaluate medication usage for cause

Second-Degree AV Block—Mobitz I or Wenckebach Phenomenon

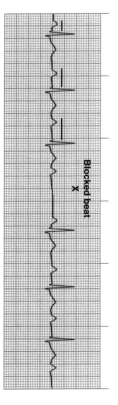

Blocked beat
X

Almost always temporary. If bradycardia → ↓ CO. Resolves when underlying condition corrected (MI, CAD, drug induced: beta blockers, calcium channel blockers).

■ ■ ■ **P wave:** Present until one P wave is blocked with no resultant QRS
■ ■ ■ **Rhythm:** Irregular
■ ■ ■ **PR interval:** Becomes progressively longer until a QRS is dropped
■ ■ ■ **QRS:** Normal
■ ■ ■ **Management:** Correct the underlying cause; atropine, temporary pacemaker; discontinue digoxin

Second-Degree AV Block—Mobitz II

Problem with bundle of His or bundle branches. Bradycardia → ↓ CO → ↓ BP. Patient symptomatic. May progress to more serious block.

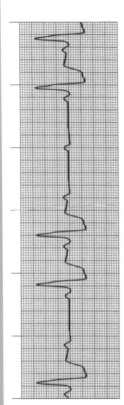

- **P wave:** Present but atrial rate > ventricular rate
  - Conduction of P waves: QRS complexes in 2:1, 3:1, or 4:1 manner
- **Rhythm:** Regular
- **PR interval:** Normal if P wave followed by QRS
- **QRS:** Normal but QRS periodically missing, sometimes wide
- **Management:** Atropine for bradycardia, isoproterenol if very slow rate, pacemaker. Consider epinephrine or dopamine as needed

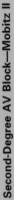

Third-Degree AV Block—Complete Heart Block

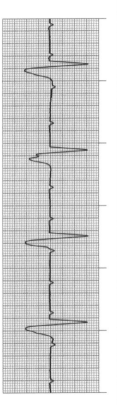

Loss of synchrony between atrial and ventricular contractions. Potentially life-threatening. Bradycardia → ↓ CO → ↓ BP. Patient symptomatic. Digoxin toxicity a frequent cause.

- **P wave:** Present but atrial rate > ventricular rate
  - Conduction of P waves in no relation to QRS complexes
- **Rhythm:** Regular atrial rate and ventricular rate
- **PR interval:** No relation of P waves to QRS complexes
- **QRS:** Usually wide
- **Management:** Atropine for bradycardia, epinephrine, isoproterenol, pacemaker

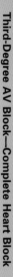

Bundle Branch Block

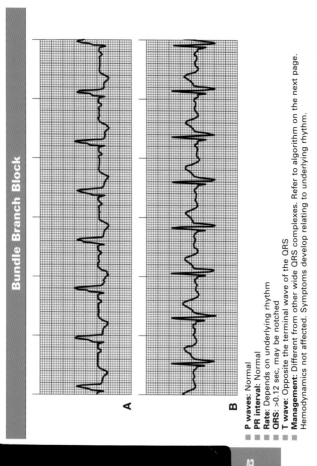

A

B

- **P waves:** Normal
- **PR interval:** Normal
- **Rate:** Depends on underlying rhythm
- **QRS:** >0.12 sec, may be notched
- **T wave:** Opposite the terminal wave of the QRS
- **Management:** Opposite from other wide QRS complexes. Refer to algorithm on the next page. Hemodynamics not affected. Symptoms develop relating to underlying rhythm.

Wide QRS Complex Tachycardia

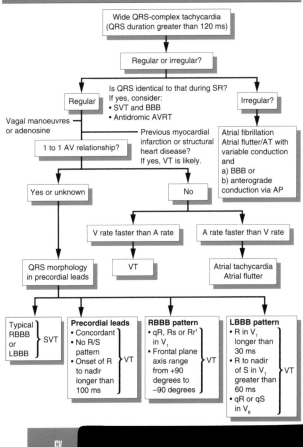

Wide QRS-complex tachycardia
(QRS duration greater than 120 ms)

Regular or irregular?

Is QRS identical to that during SR?
If yes, consider:
- SVT and BBB
- Antidromic AVRT

Regular

Irregular?

Vagal manoeuvres or adenosine

Previous myocardial infarction or structural heart disease?
If yes, VT is likely.

Atrial fibrillation
Atrial flutter/AT with variable conduction
and
a) BBB or
b) anterograde conduction via AP

1 to 1 AV relationship?

Yes or unknown

No

V rate faster than A rate

A rate faster than V rate

QRS morphology in precordial leads

VT

Atrial tachycardia
Atrial flutter

| Typical RBBB or LBBB | **Precordial leads** • Concordant • No R/S pattern • Onset of R to nadir longer than 100 ms | **RBBB pattern** • qR, Rs or Rr' in V₁ • Frontal plane axis range from +90 degrees to –90 degrees | **LBBB pattern** • R in V₁ longer than 30 ms • R to nadir of S in V₁ greater than 60 ms • qR or qS in V₆ |

Typical RBBB or LBBB } SVT

Precordial leads } VT

RBBB pattern } VT

LBBB pattern } VT

CV

Respiratory Disorders

Respiratory Failure

Respiratory failure occurs when there is either insufficient oxygenation and/or inadequate CO_2 elimination. Broadly defined as PaO_2 <50 mm Hg or $PaCO_2$ >50 mm Hg and arterial pH <7.35 when baseline ABGs are considered normal. The PaO_2/FiO_2 ratio is generally <200. Respiratory failure generally classified as either hypoxemic (type I, PaO_2 <60 mm Hg) or hypercapnic (type II, $PaCO_2$ >50 mm Hg). May also be classified as acute or chronic. Hypoxemic respiratory failure is most common type.

Clinical Presentation

■ Tachypnea, dyspnea
■ Diminished breath sounds, wheezing and rhonchi, crackles
■ Use of accessory muscles to breathe
■ Tachycardia and cardiac arrhythmias
■ Cold, clammy skin; diaphoresis
■ Ashen skin
■ Peripheral cyanosis of skin, oral mucosa, lips, and nailbeds
■ Sitting bolt upright or slightly hunched over
■ Agitation, anxiety
■ Asterixis if severe hypercapnia
■ Restlessness, lethargy, altered mental status (confused, disoriented), somnolence
■ Seizures, coma
■ Can lead to sepsis and ventilator-associated pneumonia after intubation

Diagnostic Tests

■ ABGs
■ CXR and sputum cultures
■ Pulmonary function tests
■ CBC especially WBC, Hgb, and Hct
■ ECG, echocardiogram may be helpful
■ CT scan
■ V/Q scan
■ Angiography
■ Toxicology screen
■ Serum chemistry tests

Management

■ Treat underlying cause.
■ Monitor VS, heart rhythm, fluid and electrolyte balance, intake and output.
■ Assess cardiac, respiratory, and neurological status.
■ Administer O_2 via mask or mechanical ventilation.

- Assess oxygenation: ABGs, pulse oximetry (SpO$_2$), capnography. Consider bicarbonate if acidosis present.
- Administer bronchodilators: terbutaline (Brethaire, Bricanyl), albuterol (Proventil), ipratropium bromide (Atrovent HFA).
- Administer corticosteroids: methylprednisolone (Solu-Medrol).
- Obtain blood cultures.
- Administer antibiotics if infection suspected.
- Administer analgesics for pain as indicated. Morphine if pulmonary edema present.
- Administer nitrates: nitroglycerin or nitroprusside (Nitropress), inotropes (dopamine, dobutamine, norepinephrine), and vasopressors as indicated to provide hemodynamic support.
- Provide enteral or parenteral nutritional support.
- Administer diuretics: furosemide (Lasix) or metolazone (Zaroxolyn) if refractory to Lasix.
- Consider extracorporeal membrane oxygenation (ECMO).
- Assess for complications related to mechanical ventilation (refer to Basics tab).

Acute Respiratory Distress Syndrome (ARDS)

ARDS is defined as noncardiogenic pulmonary edema characterized by severe refractory hypoxemic respiratory failure and decreased pulmonary compliance quickly leading to acute respiratory failure. May take hours or a few days.

Pathophysiology

↑ capillary/alveolar membrane permeability → interstitial and alveolar leak → right-to-left intrapulmonary shunting → severe and refractory hypoxemia, metabolic acidosis. Inactivation of surfactant → alveolar atelectasis and collapse, ↑ alveolar dead space, ↓ lung compliance, → hypoventilation and hypercapnia with severe hypoxemia.

The intrapulmonary shunt is a type of V̇/Q̇ mismatch because a percentage of cardiac output is not oxygenated as a result of collapsed or fluid-filled and nonventilated alveoli (physiological shunt), there is an absence of blood flow to already ventilated alveoli (alveoli dead space), or combination of both (refer to section on V̇/Q̇ Mismatch). In ARDS, this shunt is ≥15%.

Clinical Presentation

Symptoms of ARDS occur within 24 to 48 hr of cause and include:

- Increased respiratory rate, increased work of breathing, dyspnea, cyanosis
- Crackles, rhonchi or wheezes, dry cough
- Intercostal and suprasternal retraction, retrosternal discomfort
- Agitation, restlessness, apprehension, anxiety, confusion
- Diaphoresis
- Abdominal paradox

- Increased pressure to ventilate
- Hypoxemia refractory to increased fractional concentration of oxygen in inspired gas (FiO_2)
- Increased peak inspiratory pressure
- Decreased lung volume, decreased functional residual capacity, low V/Q ratio
- PCWP <18 mm Hg and/or no evidence of HF or left atrial hypertension
- Acute respiratory alkalosis initially, which may progress to respiratory acidosis
- Worsening ABGs with increased FiO_2, leading to marked hypoxemia, increased crackles
- Worsening PaO_2/FiO_2 ratio (P/F ratio)
- Increase in A-a gradient (difference between alveolar and arterial oxygen tension = normal value of <15 mm Hg)
- Diffuse bilateral pulmonary infiltrates on CXR indicating "whiteout"
- Fluid and electrolyte problems
- Tachycardia and arrhythmias, especially PVCs
- Labile blood pressure, hypotension
- Decreased gut motility
- Generalized edema with poor skin integrity and skin breakdown
- Symptoms of impaired coagulation
- Can lead to sepsis and ventilator-associated pneumonia after intubation

Diagnostic Tests

- ABGs and venous blood gases
- Mixed venous oxygen saturation
- Continuous oxygenation monitoring via pulse oximetry
- Pulmonary function tests
- Intrapulmonary shunt fraction is the ratio; PaO_2 to FiO_2 ratio (P/F ratio) of
  - P/F ratio >300 considered normal
  - <200 mm Hg indicative of ARDS
  - P/F ratio >200 indicative of a 15%–20% intrapulmonary shunt
  - P/F ratio >100 indicative of an intrapulmonary shunt <20%
- Pulmonary artery catheter
- Serial CXRs
- Chest CT
- ECG and echocardiogram
- CBC, metabolic panel, serum lactate (lactic acid)
- Plasma brain (B-type) natriuretic peptide (BNP) levels

Management

- Treat underlying cause. Differentiate from cardiogenic pulmonary edema.
- Administer antibiotics if infection suspected.
- Assess respiratory, cardiac, and neurological status frequently.
- Administer O_2 mask or mechanical ventilation with positive end-expiratory pressure (PEEP) or continuous positive airway pressure (CPAP) and high

FIO_2. Consider high-frequency oscillation ventilation (HFOV)—used when difficulty oxygenating a patient on conventional setting because of poor lung compliance (required neuromuscular blockade). High-flow nasal cannula or noninvasive positive-pressure ventilation (NIPPV) may be considered.

- Assess serial ABGs and pulse oximetry monitoring.
- Use ECG monitoring; assess for and treat arrhythmias. Consider pulmonary artery catheter. Values affected by intrathoracic pressure.
- Perform bedside pulmonary function testing. Consider tracheostomy if MV prolonged.
- Monitor airway pressures: mean airway pressure, peak inspiratory pressure, plateau pressure. Monitor for barotrauma, especially pneumomediastinum and/or pneumothorax.
- Provide continuous arteriovenous hemofiltration (CAVH).
- Maintain hemodynamic stability. Administer vasopressors and inotropes as indicated.
- Corticosteroids found not to be beneficial except in select cases.
- Administer bronchodilators and mucolytics. Bronchoscopy if indicated.
- Administer surfactant therapy.
- Place patient in prone position. If unable, use semi-Fowler's or high Fowler's position.
- Administer diuretic; fluid management. Administer IV fluids cautiously.
- Evaluate electrolytes, intake and output; weigh daily.
- Provide sedation or therapeutic paralysis if necessary.
- Provide pain control.
- Provide nutritional support. Consider enteral or parental feedings. Use small-bore feeding tube.
- Cluster activities to decrease fatigue.
- Institute VAP, CLABSI, and sepsis bundles of nursing care. DVT prophylaxis.
- Other management therapies for ARDS may include inhaled nitrous oxide and ECMO.
- Treatment-induced complications include:
  - Cardiac arrhythmias
  - GI bleeding, DIC, anemia
  - Malnutrition and paralytic ileus
  - Pneumothorax, pulmonary fibrosis, tracheal stenosis
  - Infections such as CLABSI, CAUTI, Clostridium difficile, MRSA, and VRE
  - ATN leading to renal failure, renal failure, multiple organ dysfunction

Extracorporeal Membrane Oxygenation (ECMO)

ECMO is a modified form of cardiorespiratory bypass. It provides oxygenation and pulmonary support for patients in severe respiratory failure, particularly ARDS. Its purpose is to avoid high oxygen concentrations and high peak inspiratory pressures, PEEP, and tidal volume, while allowing the lung to rest and heal. It can also serve as a bridge to lung transplantation. May also be used in patients with pulmonary hypertension or massive pulmonary embolism. Specific inclusion and exclusion criteria are related to its use as well as management considerations when using ECMO.

Venovenous (VV) ECMO

The right internal jugular and right common femoral veins are cannulated. The patient's blood is circulated through a membrane oxygenator in which O_2 is infused and CO_2 removed. Blood is then returned to the venous circulation via the right common femoral vein. ECMO can compensate for approximately 70% of the patient's gas exchange requirements. Provides respiratory support without hemodynamic support.

Functional oxygen saturation (Spo2) and CO_2 are monitored continuously to maintain values of 50%–80% and 35–45 mm Hg, respectively.

Complications include infections and sepsis, bleeding, DIC, intracranial bleeding, air emboli, renal failure, pressure ulcers, and heparin-induced thrombocytopenia. Nursing care focuses on maintenance of the ECMO system and prevention of complications.

Venoarterial (VA) ECMO

Blood from a large central vein is circulated through a membrane oxygenator and returned to the arterial system. VA ECMO provides both respiratory and hemodynamic support.

Ventilation/Perfusion (V/Q̇) Mismatch

Both lung capillary perfusion and alveolar ventilation are affected by body position and gravity.

- Perfusion and ventilation adequate and adequate gas exchange ← V/Q̇ match exists. Normal V/Q̇ ratio 4:5 = 0.8. If ventilation or lung capillary perfusion, or both, is not adequate ← V/Q̇ mismatch. There are several types of V/Q̇ imbalances:

  Shunting or physiological shunt (anatomical shunt, or right-to-left shunt) is defined as the flow of blood from the right side of the heart → lungs ← left side of the heart without taking part in alveolar and capillary diffusion ← pulmonary blood perfuses completely unventilated alveoli.

  - Occurs in severe ARDS, pneumonia, tumor, mucous plug, and pulmonary edema
  - A low V/Q̇ ratio exists when capillary perfusion adequate but gas exchange ineffective in the alveoli. Therefore, perfusion exceeds ventilation.
  - Dead-space V/Q̇ mismatch occurs when alveoli ventilation normal but inadequate or absent perfusion, so that adequate gas exchange is unable to occur.
  - Results from pulmonary embolism, pneumonia, pulmonary edema, ARDS, pulmonary infarction, or cardiogenic shock.

- A high V̇/Q̇ ratio exists when ventilation is normal but perfusion inadequate. Therefore, a high V̇/Q̇ ratio exists.
- An absolute shunt (true shunt, silent unit) occurs with combination of shunting and dead-space V̇/Q̇.
- Little to no perfusion and ventilation are present. This V̇/Q̇ mismatch is generally refractory to oxygen therapy.
- It is primarily caused by pneumothorax and severe ARDS.

Diagnostic Tests

- BNP and echocardiogram to rule out cardiogenic pulmonary edema
- V̇/Q̇ scan
- ABGs
- Alveolar-arterial (A-a) gradient (PAO_2/ PaO_2)
  - PAO_2 represents the partial pressure of alveolar O_2 (mm Hg).
  - PaO_2 represents the partial pressure of arterial O_2 (mm Hg).
  - Value is used to calculate the percentage of the estimated shunt.
  - Value represents the difference between the alveolar and arterial oxygen tension.
  - Normal A-a gradient value <15 mm Hg.
  - Value is increased in atrial or ventricular septal defects, pulmonary edema, ARDS, pneumothorax, and V̇/Q̇ mismatch.
- a/A ratio (PaO_2/PAO_2):
  - If ratio <0.60, shunt is worsening.
- Estimation of shunt using PaO_2/FIO_2 (P/F) ratio:
  - P/F ratio 500 indicates a 5% shunt.
  - P/F ratio 300 indicates a 15% shunt.
  - P/F ratio 200 indicates a 20% shunt.

Management

- Treatment of underlying cause and symptoms
- Continuous positive airway pressure (CPAP), PEEP, or bilevel positive airway pressure (BiPAP)

Ventilator-Associated Pneumonia (VAP)

VAP is an airway infection that develops more than 48 hr after the patient is intubated. It is associated with increased mortality, prolonged time spent on a ventilator, and increased length of ICU/hospital stay.

Pathophysiology

VAP is usually caused by gram-negative bacilli or *Staphylococcus aureus* via microaspiration of bacteria that colonize the oropharynx and upper airways or bacteria that form a biofilm on or within an endotracheal tube (ETT). The presence of an ETT also impairs cough and mucociliary clearance. Suctioning also contributes to VAP.

Clinical Presentation

VAP manifests with:

- Increased RR, HR, and temperature (>38.3°C or 101°F)
- Increased WBC (>10,000/mm³)
- Increased purulent tracheal secretions
- Crackles
- Worsening oxygenation, hypoxemia, Pao₂/Fio₂ changes

Diagnostic Tests

- CXR showing new or persistent infiltrates
- Tracheal aspirate and blood cultures
- Clinical Pulmonary Infection Score (CPIS) <6
- Bronchoscopy or bronchoalveolar lavage

Management

- Identify patients for whom noninvasive positive pressure ventilation may be more appropriate.
- Early tracheostomy has not reduced VAP incidence.
- Data are inconclusive regarding early postpyloric feeding. Feeding tubes should be placed beyond the pylorus of the stomach.
- Probiotics may be considered a preventive measure.
- Monitor for signs and symptoms of respiratory infection.
- Monitor CXR and amount and color of tracheal secretions.
- Give IV antibacterials to which the known causative bacteria are sensitive, but avoid unnecessary antibiotics. Consider:
  - Piperacillin/tazobactam (Zosyn)
  - Gentamicin (Garamycin)
  - Tobramycin (Nebcin)
  - Vancomycin (Vancocin)
  - Ceftazidime (Fortaz, Ceptaz)
  - Levofloxacin (Levaquin)
  - Imipenem/cilastatin (Primaxin)
  - Linezolid (Zyvox)
  - Ticarillin (Ticar)
  - Daptomycin (Cubicin)
  - Ticarillin (Ticar)
  - Ciprofloxacin (Cipro)
  - Amikacin (Amikin)
  - Aztreonam (Azactam)

Evidence-Based Practice 2016 Guidelines to Prevent VAP
(Ventilator Bundle)

The ideal combination of interventions is still under investigation.

- Elevate head of bed at least 30° at all times. Also consider lateral horizontal position.

- Consider continuous lateral rotation therapy (CLRT) or mechanical rotation of patients with 40° turns every 2–4 hr.
- Provide stress ulcer disease prophylaxis with H_2-receptor inhibitors.
- Provide DVT prophylaxis.
- Use meticulous hand hygiene, and use gloves appropriately. Implement and monitor strict infection control procedures before and after patient contact, contact with respiratory equipment, items in the patient's room, and contact with respiratory secretions.
- Use meticulous sterile technique when appropriate.
- Provide oral care every 12 hr, including brushing the teeth with a soft-bristle toothbrush, tap water, and toothpaste for 1–2 min; brushing the tongue. Apply lip balm and moisturizing swabs every 2–4 hr. Follow with 0.5 oz of 0.12% chlorhexidine gluconate rinse to tooth enamel, gums, and posterior oropharynx. Continue for 24 hr after extubation. Oral chlorhexidine in non–cardiac surgery patients is of questionable use.
- Use silver- or antimicrobial-coated ETTs if patient is mechanically ventilated >48 hr.
- Use a subglottic secretion drainage system (CASS). Intermittent aspiration preferred over continuous aspiration of subglottic secretions.
- Consider Mucus Shaver or Mucus Slurper to clean inner lumen of ETT of secretions and biofilm.
- Maintain ETT cuff pressures at ≥20 mm Hg. Check cuff pressures every 8 hr. Consider a pneumatic device that will maintain ETT cuff inflating pressure.
- Eliminate routine saline bronchial lavage during ETT suctioning.
- Drain condensation in ventilator tubing down and away from patient. Avoid routine changes of ventilator circuits.
- The practice of routine suctioning every 4 hr is being questioned. Do suction as needed. Replace all suction equipment every 24 hr.
- Provide "sedation vacations" at least once every 24 hr. Slowly decrease amount and frequency of sedation.
- Assess readiness to wean or extubate, and extubate as soon as possible.
- Establish spontaneous breathing trials and protocols.
- Encourage early exercise and mobility.
- Discontinue mechanical ventilation as soon as possible. Consider noninvasive ventilation (NIV) such as BiPAP and CPAP.

Pneumonia in Critical Care Patients
Hospital-Acquired Pneumonia (HAP)

Hospital-acquired pneumonia is the most common infection in ICUs. It may result from mechanical ventilation (VAP) or occurs at least 48 hr after hospitalization (nosocomial) in non-intubated patients. Refer to BAP in the Respiratory Tab.

Pathophysiology

Bacteria (gram-negative bacilli and *Staphylococcus aureus*) ← aspirated to lung → trapped by mucus-producing cells ← alveolar macrophages fail ← activation of inflammatory mediators, cellular inflation, immune activation → damage bronchial mucous membrane and alveolocapillary membrane ← fill acini and terminal bronchioles with infectious debris and exudates ← edema and impaired gas exchange. May progress to MRSA (Refer to Basics Tab) or *Pseudomonas* infections.

Clinical Presentation

HAP manifests with:

■ Rapidly rising temperature (101°F–105°F or 38.5°C–40.5°C)
■ Chest tightness or discomfort; pleuritic chest pain
■ Diaphoresis, chills, general malaise or weakness
■ Tachycardia
■ Tachypnea (25–45 breaths/min), shortness of breath (SOB), dyspnea, cough
■ Increased tracheal secretions or change in color (creamy yellow, green, or rust colored)
■ Inspiratory and expiratory crackles
■ Diminished breath sounds
■ Worsening oxygenation or increase in O_2 requirement or need for respiratory assistance

Diagnostic Tests

■ CXR showing new or progressive lung infiltrates
■ Sputum and blood cultures
■ CBC, ESR, leukocytes (<4,000/mm³ or ≥12,000/mm³, band form ≥50%
■ ABGs or Sao$_2$ (<95%)
■ Bronchoscopy or transtracheal aspiration for cultures
■ Pneumonia Severity Index (PSI/PORT) for adult CAP interactive scoring system can be found at https://www.mdcalc.com/psi-port-score-pneumonia-severity-index-cap may be useful

Management

■ Monitor CXR and amount and color of tracheal secretions.
■ Provide oxygenation and ventilation: O_2 by cannula/mask, mechanical ventilation. Assess oxygenation status by ABGs or pulse oximetry.
■ Provide adequate hydration and nutrition.
■ Administer mucolytics and encourage effective coughing and deep breathing. Provide chest physiotherapy.
■ Administer bronchodilators.
■ Change patient's position frequently to enhance clearance of secretions and improve ventilation. Place in semi-Fowler's position.

- Give antibacterials to which the known causative bacteria are sensitive. Consider:
  - Piperacillin/tazobactam (Zosyn)
  - Levofloxacin (Levaquin)
  - Imipenem/cilastatin (Primaxin)
  - Meropenem (Merrem)
  - Change or add antibiotics if MRSA (Vancomycin or Linezolid) or *Pseudomonas* (Ceftazidime or Cefepime) infections arise
  - Routine antiseptic baths for ICU patients shows no benefit in preventing HAP

Pulmonary Edema

Pulmonary edema is defined as abnormal accumulation of fluid in the alveoli, lung tissues, or airway. "Flash" pulmonary edema (FPE) is a medical emergency in which there is a sudden accumulation of fluid in the lungs. May occur following pneumonectomy, AMI, mitral or aortic regurgitation, or HF.

Pathophysiology

Inadequate LV function → blood backs up into the pulmonary venous system → ↑ pressure in the pulmonary vasculature, ↑ COP → forces intravascular fluid into alveoli and interstitial spaces of lungs → impaired gas exchange → respiratory distress.

Risk factors include:

- Excess fluid in pulmonary capillaries (e.g., HF)
- Cocaine-induced pulmonary vasoconstriction
- Leakage of pulmonary capillary membrane (e.g., ARDS, pneumonia)

Clinical Presentation

- Pink, foamy, and frothy sputum
- Cough
- Decreased cardiac output
- Tachycardia
- Weak peripheral pulses
- Capillary refill >3 seconds

Symptoms of Vasoconstriction or Impending Respiratory Failure

- Peripheral cyanosis
- Pallor, diaphoresis
- Arrhythmias
- Respiratory distress: SOB, decreased respiratory rate, crackles at lung base
- Tachypnea
- Decreased SpO_2 or PaO_2 with dyspnea
- Decreased urine output

- Lethargy, fatigue
- Anxiety, agitation, and feelings of drowning
- Change in mental status

Diagnostic Tests

- CXR, CT may be useful
- ABGs and/or pulse oximetry
- CBC to assess for anemia or sepsis
- ECG
- Plasma BNP level
  - Normal level: 34–42 pg/mL (11.0–13.6 pmol/L)
- Serum cardiac markers along with serum chemistries, BUN, and creatinine
- Two-dimensional transthoracic echocardiogram
- Transesophageal echocardiogram

Management

- Maintain sitting position if BP reading permits.
- Start IV and obtain ABGs.
- Administer O_2 of 5–6 L/min by simple face mask or 1–15 L/min by nonrebreather mask with reservoir. Consider BiPAP or CPAP. Keep SpO_2 >90%.
- Increase O_2 concentration if needed. If unable to resolve respiratory distress, persistent hypoxemia, and acidosis, intubation or mechanical ventilation is needed. Consider PEEP.
- Monitor patient with cardiac monitor and pulse oximetry. Pulmonary arterial catheter may be helpful. Assess PAP and PCWP.
- If systolic BP >100, administer nitroglycerin.
- Administer diuretics: IV furosemide (Lasix). 0.5–1 mg/kg. Restrict fluids.
- Administer morphine slowly if BP is stable. Questionable use to decrease preload.
- Administer vasodilators and/or inotropes (dopamine, dobutamine, norepinephrine, milrinone), preload (NTG, diuretics, morphine, nesiritide) or afterload agents (ACE inhibitors, nitroprusside), and contractility medications as indicated.
- Consider intra-aortic balloon pumping.
- Consider ultrafiltration if evidence of renal dysfunction or diuretic resistance.
- Treat the underlying cause.

Pulmonary Arterial Hypertension (PAH) Cor Pulmonale

PAH is defined as mean pulmonary artery pressure $(PAP_m) \geq 25$ mm Hg and PCWP ≤ 15 mm Hg as measured by cardiac catheterization, with a resultant increased pulmonary vascular resistance.

Cor pulmonale is RV hypertrophy or failure resulting from pulmonary hypertension, massive pulmonary embolism, and other pulmonary/pulmonary vascular conditions. Living at high altitudes can also cause this condition.

Pathophysiology

PAH is seen in preexisting pulmonary or cardiac disease, LVF, familial pulmonary or cardiac disease, COPD, obesity, alveolar hypoventilation, smoke inhalation, high altitude, collagen vascular disease, vasoconstriction of pulmonary bed resulting from hypoxemia or acidosis, and congenital heart disease. Idiopathic causes → primary PAH.

Hypoxemia → hypertrophy of smooth muscle in pulmonary arteries → ↑ lumen vessel size → vasoconstriction → narrow of artery vessels → resistance to blood flow → RV pumps harder to move blood across the resistance → ↑ pulmonary vascular resistance → ↑ RV workload → smooth muscle proliferated → vascular obliteration → luminal obstruction → ↑ pulmonary artery pressure and PVR → RV hypertrophy, right heart dilation → RV cardiac function → RV failure. Acute PAH → cor pulmonale and may be the result of a massive pulmonary embolism.

Clinical Presentation

- Increased mean right atrial and RV pressure, decreased cardiac index, increased PAP_m
- ECG: Increased P-wave amplitude (lead II), incomplete right bundle branch block (RBBB), tall right precordial R waves, right axis deviation, and RV strain
- Hypoxemia, central cyanosis
- Labored and painful breathing, crackles, wheezing; possible pleural effusion
- JVD, liver engorgement and hepatomegaly, ascites
- Atrial gallop, splitting of S_2 or increased S_2 intensity, S_3 or S_4, ejection click
- Tachycardia, weak pulse, heart palpitations, angina-like chest pain
- LVF: SOB, DOE, hypoventilation, tachypnea, coughing, fatigue, syncope, hypotension, decreased urinary output, decreased cardiac output, shock
- RVF: Peripheral and dependent edema, weight gain, tricuspid regurgitation, JVD, prominent heave over RV palpated
- Hoarseness if pressure on left recurrent laryngeal nerve
- Anorexia; right upper quadrant pain, epigastric distress
- Fatigue, weakness, drowsiness, restlessness, agitation, confusion

Diagnostic Tests

- Electrocardiogram showing RV hypertrophy, right axis deviation
- Two-dimensional echocardiogram with Doppler flow
- CXR or CT
- Polysomnography for PAH sleep-disordered breathing
- V̇/Q̇ scan—Contraindicated in patients with primary pulmonary hypertension
- Pulmonary angiography with right-sided heart catheterization
- Pulmonary function tests
- ABGs, CBC. Screen for thryroid abnormalities common in PAH
- Autoantibody tests, HIV, liver function tests
- B-type natriuretic peptide (BNP) and N-terminal BNP elevated in PAH.

Management

- **Therapy depends on the stage of the disease and precipitating cause of PAH.**
- Patients with PAH need to be in a center with specific pulmonologist expertise in managing the disease.
- The aims are to decrease pulmonary pressure, remove excessive fluid, and decrease the risk of clotting.
- Monitor respiratory, cardiac, and neurological status.
- Institute ECG and hemodynamic monitoring. Administer antiarrhythmics as indicated. Cardioversion or radiofrequency ablation may be needed to treat atrial fibrillation/flutter. A pulmonary artery catheter (Swan Ganz) is generally indicated.
- Provide O₂ therapy; cannula, mask, ventilator. Monitor ABGs. Avoid intubation if possible.
- Administer bronchodilators as indicated.
- Consider standby therapeutic phlebotomy if Hct < 60%.
- Maintain Hgb to minimum 10 g/dL.
- Provide low-sodium diet and fluid restrictions. Correct fluid and electrolyte and acid-base disturbances. Administer diuretics as needed.
- Complex management is needed to maintain adequate preload but avoid overfilling RV → compress LV → ↓ cardiac output.
- Treat hypotension and low cardiac output as needed.
- The use of calcium channel blockers, steroids, anticoagulation, antiplatelet drugs, and endothelin receptor antagonists have been found to be more suited for non–critically ill patients with PAH but may be considered for critically ill patients as needed. Calcium channel blockers and beta blockers should be avoided in the critically ill because they reduce cardiac function.
- Dobutamine preferred if inotropes necessary. Also use of norepinephrine preferred.
- Administer digoxin (Lanoxin) as necessary.
- Administer prostanoids: treprostinil (Remodulin, Tyvaso), epoprostenol (Flolan), iloprost (Ventavis).
- Administer endothelin-receptor antagonists: bosentan (Tracleer), sitaxsentan (Thelin), ambrisentan (Letairis).
- Administer phosphodiesterase type 5 (PDE5) inhibitors: sildenafil (Viagra), tadalafil (Cialis), vardenafil (Levitra).
- Treat pulmonary embolism with thrombolytics or anticoagulants as appropriate.
- **Surgery (optional):** atrial septostomy, pulmonary thromboendarterectomy.
- Consider ECMO as a bridge to transplantation.
- Consider lung or heart-lung transplantation because biventricular HF may develop.

Pulmonary Embolism

Pulmonary embolism is defined as an obstruction of the pulmonary artery or its branch (pulmonary vasculature) by a thrombus or thrombi (blood clot) that originates in the venous circulatory system or the right side of the heart. A V/Q mismatch → hypoxemia and intrapulmonary shunt.

Pathophysiology

Usually the result of DVT in the legs. Also femoral, popliteal, and iliac veins. Other types: air, fat especially due to long bone fractures, amniotic fluid, tumors, bone marrow, septic thrombi, vegetation on heart valves.

Risk factors include:

- Venous stasis
- Surgery (gynecological, abdominal, thoracic, orthopedic)
- Pregnancy
- Estrogen therapy (BCP, HRT)
- Obesity
- Advanced age
- Carcinomas
- Immobilization
- Trauma
- Heart failure
- Stroke
- Sepsis

Thrombus obstructs the pulmonary artery or branch → ↓ blood flow to lungs → impaired/absent gas exchange → V/Q mismatch (dead space ventilation) → platelets accumulate around thrombus → release of endotoxins → constrict regional blood vessels + bronchioles → ↑ pulmonary vascular resistance → ↑ pulmonary arterial pressure → ↓ RV work to maintain pulmonary blood flow → RVF → ↓ cardiac output → ↓ systemic blood pressure → shock. A pulmonary embolism may occur with or without pulmonary infarction; small, large, or multiple thrombi may exist.

Clinical Presentation

Symptoms, which depend on size of the thrombus and areas of the occlusion and may vary from progressive dyspnea to hemodynamic collapse, may include:

- SOB, dyspnea, tachypnea, crackles, wheezing, cyanosis
- Hypoxemia with PaO_2 <80 mm Hg and SaO_2 <95%
- Chest pain (sudden, pleuritic, sharp), angina pectoris, MI
- Cardiac arrhythmias, especially new onset of atrial fibrillation, palpitations or tachycardia, hypotension, S_3 or S_4 gallop, cardiac murmur
- Acute cor pulmonale
- Fever (>37.8°C), diaphoresis, chills

Clinical signs and symptoms of thrombophlebitis include:

- Lower extremity edema
- Leg cramps
- Nausea and vomiting
- Abdominal or flank pain
- Hemoptysis, productive cough
- Mental confusion, decreased level of consciousness, delirium in elderly patients
- Restlessness, anxiety, apprehension
- Seizures, syncope
- Major obstruction of the pulmonary artery → severe dyspnea, sudden substernal pain and signs of shock, with sudden death possible within 1 hr

Diagnostic Tests

Some diagnostic tests are used to rule out other respiratory problems rather than confirm a diagnosis of pulmonary embolism.

- CXR, CT, MRI
- ECG (tall, peaked P wave; tachycardia; atrial fibrillation; RBBB)
- Echocardiogram
- ESR, WBC
- BNP
- ABGs (low Pao₂)
- D-dimer testing
- Venous ultrasonography and impedance plethysmography
- V/Q scan
- Pulmonary angiography

Diagnostic and Prognostic Clinical Scoring Systems or Calculators

- Pulmonary Embolism Severity Index (PESI) simplified) interactive scoring system can be found at https://www.mdcalc.com/pulmonary-embolism-severity-index-pesi
- Well's Criteria for Pulmonary Embolism (PE) interactive scoring system can be found at http://www.mdcalc.com/wells-criteria-for-pulmonary-embolism-pe/
- The PERC Rule for Pulmonary Embolism interactive scoring system can be found at http://www.mdcalc.com/perc-rule-for-pulmonary-embolism/

Management

- Provide oxygen by cannula, mask, or ventilator as indicated.
- Administer heparin bolus and start heparin infusion per policy.
- Monitor PT, PTT, INR.
- Administer sodium bicarbonate if acidotic.
- Administer pain medication if needed.
- Elevate head of bed; elevate lower extremities if DVT present.
- Assess vital signs; cardiac, respiratory and neurological status frequently.
- Assess for cardiac arrhythmias.

- Administer digoxin, diuretics, and antiarrhythmics as indicated.
- Treat shock symptoms as needed with dopamine (Intropin) or dobutamine (Dobutrex).
- Prepare for embolectomy or vena cava filter.
- Administer thrombolytic drug therapy: alteplase (Activase), Reteplase (Retavase), streptokinase (Streptase), or urokinase (Kinlytic). Alteplase is preferred, followed by reteplase.
- Administer morphine to manage pain and anxiety.
- Administer inotropic agents if heart failure present.
- Prevention:
  - Enoxaparin (Lovenox) 30–40 mg daily
  - Dalteparin (Fragmin) 2,500–5,000 units preoperatively and postoperatively
  - Heparin 5,000 units every 8 hr
  - Fondaparinux (Arixtra)
  - Tinzaparin (Innohep)
  - Progression to warfarin (Coumadin) once patient is well anticoagulated or direct thrombin inhibitors and Factor Xa inhibitors: rivaroxaban (Xarelto), apixaban (Ellquis), dabigatran (Pradaxa), edoxaban (Savaysa), or betrixaban (Bevyxxa)
  - Leg exercises: dorsiflexion of the feet
  - Frequent position changes, ambulation
  - Intermittent pneumonic leg compression devices and antiembolism stockings

Carbon Monoxide (CO) Toxicity

CO poisoning or toxicity is defined as an abnormal level of CO in the bloodstream. Normal carboxyhemoglobin (COHgb) level for nonsmokers is <2%; for smokers it is 5% but may be as high as 13%.

COHgb level >60% → cardiac toxicity, neurotoxicity, systemic acidosis, respiratory arrest, death.

Pathophysiology

CO affinity for Hgb is 200–300 times that of O_2. CO binds with Hgb → ↓ O_2 binding sites → more CO binds → carboxyhemoglobin forms → CO changes structure of Hgb molecules → more difficult for O_2 to bind → ↓ O_2 to tissues → tissue ischemia and hypoxemia → acute respiratory failure, ARDS, cerebral hypoxia, end-organ dysfunction, and death.

CO as an inflammatory mediator → tissue damage with ↑ capillary leakage and edema → tracheal and bronchial constriction.

CO → ↓ activity of nitric oxide → (1) peripheral vasodilation → ↓ cerebral blood flow and systemic hypotension; (2) formation of free radicals → endothelial damage and oxidative damage to brain; myocardial depression and arrhythmias → ↓ cardiac output → impaired tissue perfusion.

Clinical Presentation

Early signs: patient may appear intoxicated:

- COHgb saturation of ≤10% possible with no symptoms
- Headache, nausea, and vomiting with COHgb of ≥20%
- Diarrhea
- General fatigue, weakness
- Difficulty staying focused, dizziness
- Flu-like symptoms

Later signs:

- Chest pain, palpitations
- Dysrhythmias
- MI
- Pulmonary edema
- Throbbing headache, weakness, fatigue, dizziness, memory loss, ataxia, gait disturbances, confusion, inability to concentrate
- Skin pale to reddish purple (not a reliable sign; "When you're red, you're dead.")
- Blurred vision, retinal hemorrhages
- Tachypnea, dyspnea, respiratory alkalosis
- Nausea, vomiting, lactic acidosis, rhabdomyolysis
- Fecal and urinary incontinence
- Upper airway obstruction: hoarseness, dry cough, DOE or labored breathing, stridor, difficulty swallowing
- Brassy cough with carbonaceous (soot or carbon) sputum
- Wheezing, bronchospasm
- Hallucinations, seizures, syncope, coma when COHgb ≥40%
- Death possible if COHgb ≥60%

Diagnostic Tests

Diagnostic testing is done not only to confirm the diagnosis of CO toxicity but also to determine complications.

- COHgb and myoglobin concentration, methemoglobin
- ABG (pulse oximetry SpO_2 inaccurate)
- CO oximetry of an ABG sample or bedside pulse CO oximetry
- ECG, CXR
- CT to rule out cerebral edema and focal lesions
- Troponin, CK, CK-MB, myoglobin
- CBC and serum chemistry tests including electrolytes, glucose, BUN, creatinine, and liver function tests
- Urinalysis
- Toxicology screen, ethanol level, and cyanide levels possibly ordered
- Fiberoptic bronchoscopy and V/Q scan

Management

- Assess respiratory and neurological status.
- Monitor COHgb levels until <10%.
- Administer 100% O_2 via rebreather mask or ETT (mechanical ventilation) to increase PaO_2 levels and decrease $PaCO_2$ levels. Pulse oximetry not valid.
- Assess LOC using Glasgow Coma Scale.
- Monitor pH level if lactic acidosis present.
- Monitor cardiac status. Myocardial injury is a common consequence of moderate to severe CO poisoning → higher risk of death. Monitor for arrhythmias.
- Administer hyperbaric O_2 therapy within 2–6 hr after exposure if symptoms are severe or if COHgb levels ≥25%.
- Provide supportive care.

Pneumothorax

Pneumothorax is defined as air entering the pleural space and interrupting the negative pressure, with resulting partial or total lung collapse.

Types of pneumothorax include:

- **Spontaneous pneumothorax:** Rupture of subpleural bleb with unknown cause that may be related to smoking and connective tissue disorder. Patients with chronic lung disease (COPD) have a higher incidence.
- **Traumatic pneumothorax:** Caused by blunt chest trauma, penetrating injury, pulmonary contusion → rib fracture or puncture directly to the lung → penetrates parietal and visceral pleura → punctures the lung parenchyma → lung air pressure from positive to negative pressure environment (inside the lung) → pneumothorax. If pneumothorax remains confined → ↑ air in pleural space on inspiration → air cannot exit on expiration → pressure ↑.
- **Tension pneumothorax:** Resulting from increased pressure in the pleural space that causes the lung to collapse. The increase in pressure may impair circulation by compressing the heart and vena cava.

Pneumothorax can also be categorized by size:

- Small pneumothorax (<15%)
- Moderate pneumothorax (15%–60%)
- Large pneumothorax (>60%)

Clinical Presentation

Pneumothorax manifests with:

- Respiratory distress, including shortness of breath, dyspnea, or air hunger
- Use of accessory muscles
- Anxiety

- Sharp pleuritic chest pain that increases with deep inspiration or chest movement and cough on the ipsilateral side, with pain possibly radiating to the shoulder, neck, or epigastrium
- Decreased or absent breath sounds, hyperresonance to percussion, absent tactile fremitus on the affected side, asymmetrical chest wall movement
- Hypoxemia, decreased oxygenation levels
- Cool, clammy skin or central cyanosis if hypoxemia severe
- Tachycardia, hypotension
- Subcutaneous emphysema → swelling in affected area with crepitus upon auscultation

Can develop into tension pneumothorax → severe respiratory distress, cyanosis, absent breath sounds on the affected side, sinus tachycardia >140 bpm, JVD → tracheal deviation → midline shift, hypotension, changes in mental status.

Diagnostic Tests

- CXR
- ABGs
- CT scan
- ECG

Management

- Assess vital signs, skin color, breathing pattern, breath sounds, pain level, and oxygenation.
- Assess for arrhythmias.
- Keep patient upright.
- Administer O_2 as needed by nasal cannula or mask, and monitor O_2 saturation.
- Administer analgesics as needed.
- Insert chest tube (refer to section on Chest Tubes).
- In the case of a small pneumothorax (usually <30%), no symptoms, and uncomplicated), observe and monitor the patient for pneumothorax resolution at 1.25% every day.

Thoracic Procedures

Thoracic Surgery

Segmental resection is the removal of the bronchus, a portion of the pulmonary artery and vein, and tissue of the involved lung segment.

Lobectomy is the removal of an entire lobe of the lung.

Pneumonectomy is the removal of the entire lung, generally for treatment of lung cancer, bronchiectasis, tuberculosis, or lung abscess. Removal of the right lung is more dangerous because of its larger vascular bed.

Management
Pneumonectomy (Postoperative; First 24–48 Hours)
■ Routine postoperative care includes frequent assessments of cardio-pulmonary and hemodynamic status.
■ Patient should lie on back or operative side only. This prevents leaking of bronchial stump, prevents fluid from draining into operative site, and allows full expansion of remaining lung.
■ Perform CXR to check for deviation of trachea from midline indicating mediastinal shift.
■ Patient may need chest tube or thoracostomy needle aspiration.
■ Provide routine nursing care related to chest tubes (refer to section on Chest Tubes). Avoid connecting chest tube to wall suction. Chest tube is connected to gravity drainage only.
■ Assess for signs and symptoms: neck vein distention, ↑ HR, ↑ RR, dyspnea, trachea displaced to one side.
■ Note that remaining lung needs 2–4 days to adjust to increased blood flow.
■ Monitor fluid and electrolyte balance to prevent fluid overload (e.g., crackles, increased HR, increased BP, dyspnea). Administer IV fluids with caution to prevent fluid overload and pulmonary edema.
■ Provide O_2 therapy. Mechanical ventilation may be needed; monitor level of oxygenation. Administer pulmonary function tests, such as forced expiratory volume (volume of air patient can forcibly exhale after a full inspiration). Monitor respiratory and oxygenation status.
■ Encourage coughing, deep breathing, and splinting.
■ Elevate head of bed 30°–45°.
■ Administer analgesia as needed.
■ Monitor ECG to detect cardiac arrhythmias, especially atrial arrhythmias.
■ Monitor vital signs to detect hypotension.
■ Monitor for pulmonary edema and subcutaneous emphysema.

Complications of Pneumonectomy
■ Atelectasis, pneumonia, tension pneumothorax, empyema, bronchopleural fistula (increased temperature, cough, increased WBC, anorexia, purulent sputum)
■ Excessive blood loss, hemorrhage
■ Respiratory distress and pulmonary edema
■ Cardiac dysrhythmias and hypotension

Chest Tubes

A chest tube is inserted into the pleural space to reestablish negative intrapleural pressure or to remove air, fluid, or blood. It is inserted after cardiac surgery, if needed, and to treat pneumothorax, hemothorax, empyema, or pleural effusion. It may also be used for intrapleural administration of chemotherapeutic agents or a mechanical agent (talc slurry).

RESP

A mediastinal tube is inserted into the mediastinal space to provide fluid and bloody drainage after cardiac surgery to prevent tamponade. It is managed the same as a chest tube.

A three-chamber water system or dry suction (waterless) is generally used.

- Three-chamber system has water seal, drainage, and suction chambers.
- Dry suction has only water seal and drainage chambers. Can provide higher levels of suction, easier to set up and manage, quiet, and absence of water evaporation.
- Heimlich valves (one-way flutter valves) are used in the outpatient and ED setting or by emergency medical providers in the field.

Management

- Perform CXR immediately after insertion and every day thereafter.
- Apply sterile occlusive gauze dressing to the chest tube site. Change dressing as per institutional policy.
- Attach chest tube to water seal drainage; use wall suction or gravity as indicated.
- Suction control chamber should be set to 20 cm H_2O level. Fluid level regulates amount of suction → low → add sterile water to chamber.
- Wall suction is contraindicated after pneumonectomy.
- Bubbling should be constant but gentle → "slow boil."
- Monitor vital signs every 15 min until stable, then every 4 hr.
- Monitor color, amount, and consistency of drainage every 2 hr. Notify physician if drainage >100–200 mL/hr or if sudden change in drainage characteristics. Progress to every 8 hr.
- Administer O_2 via nasal cannula or mask; monitor oxygenation levels.
- Medicate for pain as needed.
- Reposition patient every 2 hr.
- Make sure all connections are tight.
- Avoid dependent loops, kinks, or pressure in tubing.
- Keep drainage system below the level of the chest.
- Palpate for subcutaneous emphysema or crepitus around insertion site and chest wall. Assess for air leak around insertion site and within chest drainage system.
- Signs of air leak may include bubbles in water seal chamber during inspiration, coughing, and large area of subcutaneous emphysema. Locate source of air leak by gently pinching chest tube near insertion site. If bubbling stops → leak is at the insertion site or inside the patient. If bubbling persists → leak in the system → replace chest tube, retape connections, or replace drainage system.
- Auscultate breath sounds; assess respirations.
- Observe color and consistency of drainage; mark fluid level of drainage
- Check water seal level; add sterile water if needed.
- Avoid clamping the chest tube as it can lead to tension pneumothorax.
- Never clamp the chest tube to transport the patient.

■ Change drainage system if significant air leak in the system or if drainage chambers full. Double clamp chest tube close to the insertion site with two clamps facing in opposite directions. Never leave chest tube clamped for more than 1 min.

Complications:

■ Rapid and shallow breathing
■ Cyanosis
■ Hemorrhage
■ Significant changes in vital signs
■ Increased subcutaneous emphysema

Chest tube removal (when there is no air leak for 24 hr, drainage <100 mL/day, and CXR shows almost complete lung expansion):

■ Premedicate with analgesics ½ hr before removal.
■ Place patient in semi-Fowler's position.
■ Use Vaseline gauze on a sterile dressing and hold over chest tube site. Have patient take a deep breath and perform Valsalva maneuver during expiration → chest tube is removed while rapidly covering the chest tube insertion site with the gauzed dressing.
■ Perform follow-up CXR.

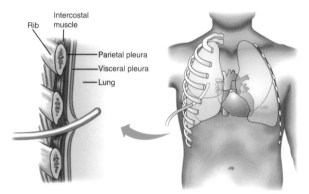

Chest tube placement between ribs and pleural space of lung.

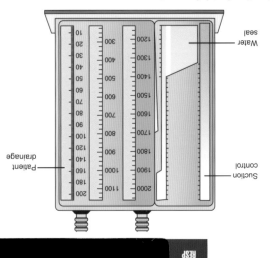

Wet suction chest drainage system.

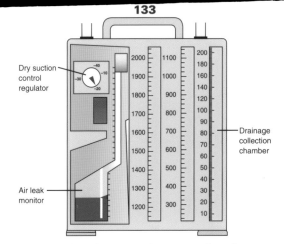

Dry suction control regulator

Air leak monitor

Drainage collection chamber

Dry suction chest tube drainage system (most commonly used).

Acute Kidney Injury (AKI)

- Acute kidney injury (AKI) was previously referred to as acute renal failure (ARF).
- AKI is a clinical syndrome characterized by rapid decline in renal function (within 48 hr) → progressive azotemia and ↑ creatinine. It is associated with oliguria, which can progress over hours or days with ↑ in BUN, creatinine, and K⁺ with or without oliguria. It is usually reversible.
- Chronic kidney disease develops slowly over months to years and necessitates the initiation of dialysis or transplantation. Chronic kidney disease is not a critical care issue. Although it is seen regularly in an ICU setting, it is generally not the reason for admission to the ICU.

Pathophysiology

The three primary causes of AKI are:

- **Prerenal failure:** Caused by renal hypoperfusion conditions such as hemorrhage, myocardial infarction, heart failure, cardiogenic shock, sepsis, and anaphylaxis → impaired blood flow to kidneys → hypoperfusion of kidneys → retention of excessive amount of nitrogenous compounds → intense vasoconstriction → ↓ GFR. Patient can recover if fluid is replaced. Most common cause of AKI.
- **Intrarenal failure:** Caused by burns, crush injuries, infections, glomerulonephritis, lupus erythematosus, diabetes mellitus, malignant HTN, nephrotoxic agents → acute tubular necrosis → afferent arteriole vasoconstriction → hypoperfusion of the glomerular apparatus → ↑ GFR → obstruction of tubular lumen by debris and casts, interstitial edema, or release of intrarenal vasoactive substances. Nonrecovery is common.
- **Postrenal failure:** Caused by any obstruction to urine flow such as bladder tumors, renal calculi, enlarged prostate, or blocked catheter between the kidneys and urethral meatus → ↑ pressure in kidney tubules → ↑ GFR.

Risk Factors for AKI

- Triple therapy using an anti-inflammatory drug (NSAID) combined with two antihypertensive medications (a diuretic plus an ACE inhibitor or angiotensin-receptor blocker) significantly increases the risk for AKI.
- Nephrotoxic drugs include chemotherapeutic agents, heavy metals, radiocontrast agents and drugs such as vancomycin, NSAIDs, fluoxetine (Prozac), lithium, benzodiazepines, among others.

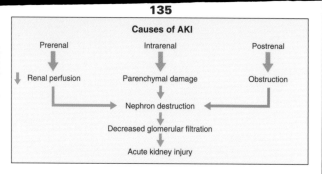

Causes of AKI

Prerenal	Intrarenal	Postrenal
↓ Renal perfusion	Parenchymal damage	Obstruction

→ Nephron destruction ←

Decreased glomerular filtration

Acute kidney injury

Risk Injury Failure Loss End-Stage (RIFLE) Classification System for AKI Consists of Three Stages and Two Outcome Measures

Stage	GFR or Serum Creatinine Criteria	Urine Output Criteria
Risk Stage 1	GFR decrease >25% baseline or Serum creatinine increased · 1.5 baseline	Urine output <0.5 mL/kg/hr for 6 hr
Injury Stage 2	GFR decrease >50% baseline or Serum creatinine increased · 2 baseline	Urine output <0.5 mL/kg/hr for 12 hr
Failure Stage 3	GFR decrease >75% baseline or Serum creatinine increased × 3 baseline or creatinine >4 mg/dL; acute rise >0.5 mg/dL	Urine output <0.3 mL/kg/hr for 24 hr or anuria for 12 hr
Loss	Complete loss of renal function >4 wk	
End-stage kidney disease (ESKD)	Complete loss of renal function >3 mo	

Patients can be classified by GFR criteria or urine output criteria, but criteria that support the most severe classification should be used.

Clinical Presentation

AKI manifests as:

- Critical illness
- Lethargy
- Persistent nausea and vomiting
- Diarrhea
- Dry skin and mucous membranes from dehydration
- Drowsiness
- Headache
- Muscle twitching
- Seizures
- Heart failure
- Liver disease

Signs of AKI include:

- Urine <400 mL/24 hr; hematuria may or may not be present
- ↓ serum urea and creatinine
- Peripheral and systemic edema, JVD, weight gain, ascites
- ↑ BP ← fluid overload ← pulmonary and peripheral edema
- ↑ BP ← dehydration and dry mucous membranes, flat JVD
- Tachycardia, abnormal and irregular pulse → cardiac arrhythmia
- Kussmaul's respirations ← metabolic acidosis
- ↓ temperature ← infection; sepsis
- ↑ LOC, lethargy, coma, seizures
- Electrolyte imbalance (increased serum BUN, creatinine, K⁺, Na⁺, phosphate; decreased serum calcium)
- High bladder pressures: patients with bladder pressures > 25 mm Hg suspected of having AKI from abdominal compartment syndrome

Diagnostic Tests

- Serum BUN, creatinine, BUN/Cr ratio, electrolytes, CBC, coagulation studies (PT/PTT), serum osmolarity, chemistry panel, total protein, albumin, uric acid
- Fractional excretion of Na (FENa) and urea (FEUrea)
- Urinalysis with microscopic examination for protein and casts
- Urine culture and sensitivity
- Urine electrolytes, urine creatinine, specific gravity, and urine osmolarity
- 24-hr urine for creatinine clearance
- ECG
- Renal ultrasound scanning
- ABGs and CXR

- Renal biopsy
- GFR rate
- Kidney-ureters-bladder (KUB) x-ray, intravenous pyelogram (IVP), excretory urography, nephrotomography
- CT scan or MRI of kidneys
- Renal angiography

Management

- Monitor and correct fluid and electrolyte imbalances.
- Assess and correct acid-base imbalances. Consider administering bicarbonate.
- Assess respiratory status and monitor oxygenation. Administer O_2 as indicated.
- Institute cardiac monitor, and observe for arrhythmias.
- Restrict fluid intake, and measure intake and output strictly. Assess for edema.
- Assess color and clarity of urine output. Check specific gravity.
- Institute renal diet with adequate protein and low K^+, Na^+, and phosphorus. Protein may be restricted if BUN and creatinine greatly elevated. Dietary consult.
- Treat anorexia, nausea, and vomiting.
- Monitor daily weight.
- Insert a large-bore central line.
- Administer medications, including antihypertensives, calcium channel blockers, beta blockers, and diuretics such as bumetanide (Bumex) and furosemide (Lasix). Administer meds cautiously in patients with impaired renal function.
- Administer iron supplement or recombinant human erythropoietin (Epogen).
- Monitor hemoglobin and hematocrit levels for anemia and O_2-carrying capacity of hemoglobin. Administer blood products as needed.
- Maintain meticulous skin care to prevent skin breakdown.
- Ensure prevention of secondary infections.
- Assess for gastrointestinal and cutaneous bleeding.
- Assess neurological status for changes in LOC and confusion.
- Administer dialysis (hemodialysis, peritoneal dialysis, or continuous renal replacement therapy [CRRT]).
- Provide patient and family support.

60

Treatment of Renal Disorders

Renal Replacement Therapy

Renal replacement therapy (RRT) is a general term used to describe the various substitution treatments available for severe, acute, and end-stage chronic renal failure (ESCRF), including dialysis (hemodialysis and peritoneal dialysis), hemo-filtration, and renal transplant. Peritoneal dialysis is generally not recommended in critically ill patients. Research has shown that CRRT and hemodialysis improve patient outcomes better than peritoneal dialysis in this population.

Hemodialysis

Hemodialysis is one of several RRTs used in the treatment of renal failure to remove excess fluids and waste products → restores chemical and electrolyte imbalances.

Pathophysiology

Hemodialysis involves passing the patient's blood through an artificial semiper-meable membrane to perform filtering and excretion functions that the kidney can no longer do effectively.

Procedure

Dialysis works by using passive transfer of toxins by diffusion (movement of molecules from an area of higher concentration to an area of lower concentration). Blood and dialysate (dialyzing solution) containing electrolytes and H_2O (closely resembling plasma) flow in opposite directions through the semipermeable membrane. The patient's blood contains excess H_2O and excess electrolyte and metabolic waste. During dialysis, the waste products and excess H_2O move from blood → dialysate because of the differences in concentrations. Electrolytes can move in or out of blood or dialysate. This circulating pattern takes place over a preset length of time, generally 3–4 hr.

Components

The components of the hemodialysis system include:

■ Dialyzer
■ Dialysate
■ Vascular access: subclavian vein, arteriovenous fistula or graft, femoral vein
■ Hemodialysis machine

Heparin is used to prevent blood clots from forming in the dialyzer or in the blood tubing. The heparin dose is adjusted to the patient's needs.

Hemodialysis Nursing Care

■ Obtain baseline VS and SpO_2 via pulse oximetry.
■ Obtain baseline weight. Assess for edema and JVD.
■ Assess breath and heart sounds.

- Monitor ECG for arrhythmias.
- Assess for disequilibrium syndrome: restlessness, ↓ LOC, headache, muscle twitching, and seizures, and stop dialysis if necessary.
- Many drugs are dialyzable. Medications may be held during dialysis.
- Vasoactive drugs can cause hypotension → may be held until after dialysis.
- Antibiotics may be given after dialysis and administered on days patients receive dialysis.

Postdialysis Care

- Monitor vital signs every hour × 4 hr, then every 4 hr (hypotension may occur secondary to hypovolemia thus requiring IV fluids; ↑ temperature may occur after dialysis secondary to blood warming mechanism of the hemodialysis machine).
- Weigh after dialysis.
- Monitor vascular access site for bleeding.
- Assess fistula or graft for bruit and thrill ("hear the bruit and feel the thrill").
- Avoid all invasive procedures for 4–6 hr after dialysis if anticoagulation used.

Continuous Renal Replacement Therapy (CRRT)

CRRT represents a family of modalities that provides continuous support of severely ill patients in AKI. It is used when hemodialysis is not feasible. CRRT works more slowly than hemodialysis and requires continuous monitoring. It is indicated for patients who are no longer responding to diuretic therapy, are in fluid overload, and/or are hemodynamically unstable.

Procedure

CRRT requires placement of a continuous arteriovenous hemofiltration (CAVH) catheter or continuous venovenous hemofiltration (CVVH) catheter and a mean arterial pressure of 60 mm Hg.

Other types of CRRT include:

- Continuous arteriovenous hemodialysis (CAVHD)
- Continuous venovenous hemodialysis (CVVHD)
- Slow continuous ultrafiltration (SCUF)
- Continuous arteriovenous hemodiafiltration (CAVHDF)
- Continuous venovenous hemodiafiltration (CVVHDF)

Because it is difficult to obtain and maintain arterial access, CVVH or venous access is preferred.

CRRT provides for the removal of fluid, electrolytes, and solutes.

CRRT differs from hemodialysis in the following ways:

- It is continuous rather than intermittent, and large fluid volumes can be removed over days instead of hours.
- Intermittent renal replacement therapy (IRRT) is a variation of CRRT and may be an option for select patients.

- Solute removal can occur by convection (no dialysate required), in addition to osmosis and diffusion.
- It causes less hemodynamic instability.
- It requires a trained ICU RN to care for patient but does not require constant monitoring by a specialized hemodialysis nurse.
- It does not require hemodialysis equipment, but a modified blood pump is required.
- It is the ideal treatment for someone who needs fluid and solute control but cannot tolerate rapid fluid removal.
- It can be administered continuously, for as long as 30–40 days. The hemofilter is changed every 24–48 hr or per policy.

Nursing Care
- Monitor fluid and electrolyte balance including intake and output.
- Weigh daily.
- Monitor vital signs every hour. A fever may be masked by the continuous cool fluids circulating. Assess Spo₂ by pulse oximetry as needed.
- Perform ECG monitoring.
- Assess and provide care of vascular access site every shift.

Complications
- Electrolyte and pH imbalances
- Hypotension
- Increased blood glucose levels
- Hypothermia
- Clogged filters

Renal Transplant

A renal transplant is the surgical placement of a cadaveric kidney or live donor kidney (including all arterial and venous vessels and long piece of ureter) into a patient with end-stage renal disease (ESKD).

Operative Procedure

The surgical procedure takes 4–5 hr. The transplanted kidney is usually placed in the right iliac fossa to allow for easier access to the renal artery, vein, and ureter attachment. The patient's nonfunctioning kidney usually stays in place unless concern exists about chronic infection in one or both kidneys. Renal transplants may be done in conjunction with pancreatic transplants.

Postoperative Care
- Monitor vital signs as per policy. Note signs and symptoms of infection.
- Monitor hourly urine output, and assess urine color. Strict intake and output. Provide meticulous Foley catheter care.

- Obtain daily urinalysis, urine electrolytes, urine for acetones, and urine culture and sensitivity.
- Administer immunosuppressive drug therapy (↑ risk of infection). These may include glucocorticosteroids, cyclosporine, tacrolimus.
- Monitor daily weight.
- Administer IV fluids cautiously.
- Administer diuretics as needed.
- Obtain daily basic metabolic panel (BMP). Assess electrolytes, BUN, creatinine, osmolarity, CBC.

Institution-Specific Care:

- _____
- _____
- _____
- _____
- _____

Complications

- Rejection (most common and serious complication): A reaction between the antigens in the transplanted kidney and the antibodies in the recipient's blood → tissue destruction → kidney necrosis. Rejection can occur at any time from immediately to many years later.
- Thrombosis to the major renal artery may occur up to 2–3 days post-op → may be indicated by sudden ↓ in urine output → emergency surgery is required to prevent ischemia to the kidney.
- Renal artery stenosis → HTN is the manifestation of this complication → a bruit over the graft site or ↓ in renal function may be other indicators → may be repaired surgically or by balloon angioplasty.
- Vascular leakage or thrombosis → requires emergency nephrectomy surgery.
- Wound complications: hematomas, abscesses → ↑ risk of infection → exertion on new kidney. Infection is major cause of death in transplant recipient. These patients are on immunosuppressive therapy → signs and symptoms of infection may not manifest in the usual way. Watch for low-grade fevers, mental status changes, and vague complaints of discomfort.

Radical Nephrectomy

Radical nephrectomy is the removal of the kidney; the ipsilateral adrenal gland; surrounding tissue; and, at times, surrounding lymph nodes. Because of the increased risk of recurrence in the ureteral stump, ureterectomy may be performed as well.

Pathophysiology

Primary indication is for treatment of renal cell carcinoma (adenocarcinoma of the kidney), in which the healthy tissue of the kidney is destroyed and replaced by cancer cells.

Secondary indication is for treatment of renal trauma → penetrating wounds or blunt injuries to back, flank, or abdomen injuring the kidney; injury or laceration to the renal artery → hemorrhage.

Clinical Presentation

- Flank pain (dull, aching)
- Gross hematuria
- Palpable renal mass
- Abdominal discomfort or pain (present in 5%–10% of cases)
- Hematuria (late sign)
- Muscle wasting, weakness, poor nutritional status, weight loss (late signs)

Diagnostic Tests

- Urinalysis (may show RBCs)
- CBC
- Complete metabolic panel (CMP)
- ESR (sed rate)
- Human chorionic gonadotropin (hCG) level
- Cortisol level
- Adrenocorticotropic hormone level
- Renin level
- Parathyroid hormone level
- Cystoscopy
- IV urogram
- Renal angiogram or nephrotomogram
- Ultrasound, CT of abdomen/pelvis with contrast
- MRI, MRA

Postoperative Management

- Monitor vital signs frequently.
- Provide pain management.
- Encourage patient to cough and deep breathe and to use incentive spirometer every hour.
- Encourage early mobilization.
- Monitor intake and output strictly.
- Assess for bleeding.
- Administer IV fluids.
- May require blood transfusion.
- Obtain CBC every 6 hr × 24 hr, then every 12 hr for 24 hr early post-op.
- Monitor daily weight.
- Monitor for adrenal insufficiency.
- If drain in place, monitor and record color and amount of drainage.

Cystectomy

Radical cystectomy is the removal of the bladder, prostate, and seminal vesicles in men and the bladder, ureters, cervix, urethra, and ovaries in women. The ureters are diverted into collection reservoirs → urinary diversion (ileal conduit, continent pouch, bladder reconstruction [neobladder], ureterosigmoidostomy).

Pathophysiology

Primary indication is for treatment of carcinoma of the bladder (transitional cell, squamous cell, or adenocarcinoma). Once the cancer spreads beyond the transitional cell layer, the risk of metastasis ↑ greatly.

Secondary indication is as part of pelvic exenteration for sarcomas or tumors of the GI tract or gynecological system.

Clinical Presentation

- Gross painless hematuria (chronic or intermittent)
- Bladder irritability with dysuria, urgency, and frequency
- Urine cytology positive for neoplastic or atypical cells
- Urine tests positive for bladder tumor antigens
- Incidental or symptomatic obstructive hydroureteronephrosis

Diagnostic Tests

- Urine cytology
- Urine for bladder tumor antigens
- IV pyelogram or retrograde ureteropyelography of bladder
- Ultrasound of bladder, kidneys, and ureters
- CT of abdomen and pelvis
- MRI of abdomen and pelvis
- Cystoscopy and biopsy (confirmation of bladder carcinoma)
- Bladder barbotage (bladder washings) for cytology

Postoperative Management

- Provide routine postoperative care.
- Monitor vital signs per hospital policy immediately postoperatively.
- Encourage patient to cough and deep breathe and to use incentive spirometer every hour.
- Monitor and record amount of bleeding from incision and in urine.
- Monitor and record intake and output.
- If patient has a cutaneous urinary diversion, assess stoma for warmth and color every 8 hr in early post-op period (ostomy appliance will collect urine).
- Collaborate with enteral stoma nurse regarding stoma, skin, and urinary drainage.
- If Penrose drain or plastic catheters in place, monitor and record drainage.
- Monitor hemoglobin and hematocrit levels.
- Provide pain management.
- Encourage early ambulation.
- Provide patient and family support.

Increased Intracranial Pressure (ICP)

Increased ICP is an increase in pressure on the brain within the cranium or skull caused by an increase in cerebrospinal fluid (CSF) pressure. Normal ICP is 1–10 mm Hg with an upper limit of 15 mm Hg. Sustained ICP < 60 mm Hg is usually fatal.

Cerebral perfusion pressure (CPP) is a function of the mean arterial pressure (MAP) and ICP. If the CPP drops to <80 mm Hg, ischemia may occur. A minimum of 50 mm Hg is needed for brain perfusion; brain death occurs if perfusion pressure <30 mm Hg.

CPP should be maintained at 70–90 or 80–100 mm Hg and the ICP at <15 mm Hg.

CPP = MAP − ICP.

MAP = systolic blood pressure (SBP) + 2 (diastolic blood pressure [DBP]) ÷ 3.

Pathophysiology

- Risk factor → ↑ intracranial volume of CSF → ↑ ICP → ↓ cerebral perfusion, ↑ brain swelling, cerebral edema → a shift in brain tissue through the dura → herniation → death. Increased ICP also leads to brain tissue ischemia/ infarction and brain death.

- Herniation results in a downward shifting of brain tissue from an area of high pressure to low pressure, usually into the brainstem → coma and death.

Clinical Presentation

- Slow, bounding pulse and irregular respirations. Widening pulse pressure, especially with bradycardia, and increased BP, is highly indicative of elevated ICP.

- Decreased level of consciousness (LOC) with increasing ICP: headache and changes in LOC, slow speech, restlessness, anxiety, confusion, ↑ drowsiness, inability to be aroused.

- Stupor, coma, decortication, decerebration, and flaccidity.

- Sluggishly reactive pupils ← fixed and dilated ("blown pupils"). May be unequal.

- Blurred vision, photophobia.

- Nausea and vomiting.

- Respiratory impairment (Cheyne-Stokes), irregular or absence of breathing → death.

- Cushing's triad or response/reflex: ↑↑ cerebral blood flow → cerebral ischemia → ↑ arterial pressure and ↑ SBP, bradypnea, widening pulse pressure and reflex bradycardia (late sign). Changes in VS are late signs.

Decerebrate Position

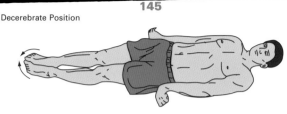

Decorticate Position

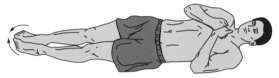

Complications

- Brainstem herniation, brain anoxia, death
- Diabetes insipidus
- SIADH

Diagnostic Tests

- Serum electrolytes and serum osmolarity
- Cerebral angiography, CT scan, MRI, PET to rule out physiological cause
- Transcranial doppler (TCD) studies
- Avoid lumbar puncture; can lead to brain herniation
- ICP monitoring devices: ventricular drainage, intracranial bolts, intraparenchymal fiberoptic catheter

Management

- Treatment is based on trends and sustained elevations of ICP and low CPP. Goal is to maintain MAP >90 mm Hg and CPP >70 mm Hg.
- Administer osmotic diuretic (mannitol [Osmitrol] 0.25–1 g/kg). Refer to hospital policy for administration procedures. Restrict fluids if necessary.
- Administer diuretics such as furosemide (Lasix).
- Insert Foley catheter to monitor output. Monitor fluid intake.

NEURO

- Monitor serum electrolytes and osmolarity.
- Administer IV hypertonic saline (>0.9% NaCl). Administer fluid boluses only with hypertonic or isotonic fluids. Avoid hypotonic dextrose solutions.
- Institute mechanical ventilation according to ABGs.
- Maintain patent airway, suction cautiously (can ↓ ICP), oxygenate, and avoid PEEP (can ↑ ICP).
- Assess respiratory status, and monitor ABGs and oxygenation.
- Use caution when suctioning patients. Hyperventilation maneuvers or aggressive "bagging" no longer recommended for initial treatment. Hyperventilation increases metabolic demand and can increase ICP.
- Monitor jugular venous oxygen saturation (SjO₂) = 55%–70% to assess O₂ content of cerebral venous blood.
- Monitor brain tissue oxygenation (PbtO₂) to assess cerebral ischemia and hypoxia. Recommended level >20.
- Consider neuromuscular blocking agents: pancuronium, atracurium, cisatracurium.
- Assess neurological and mental status by Glasgow Coma Scale or FOUR Score coma scale, including reflexes, pupils, motor and sensory function, and cranial nerve function (extraocular movements, peripheral facial droop, tongue deviation, gag reflex, corneal reflex, doll's eyes).
- Assess for meningeal signs such as headache, nuchal (neck) rigidity, photophobia
- Assess response to verbal and painful stimuli.
- Monitor vital signs, CPP, and ICP, and control fever with antipyretics. Avoid shivering, which ↑ ICP. For every 1°C rise in body temperature ← 5%–6% ↑ cerebral blood flow.
- Consider therapeutic hypothermia to ↓ cerebral edema. Hypothermia use is controversial.
- Keep head in midline position (HOB 30°–60°).
- Avoid extreme rotation of neck and neck flexion.
- Avoid extreme hip flexion.
- Monitor serum glucose and administer insulin as indicated as metabolic changes may occur. Provide enteral nutrition. Avoid aspiration.
- Monitor and treat cardiac dysrhythmias and prolongation of QT interval.
- Administer stool softeners to avoid straining at stool and prevent Valsalva maneuver.
- Maintain cardiac output using inotropes such as dobutamine (Dobutrex) and norepinephrine (Levophed)
- Administer IV sedation cautiously. Consider midazolam (Versed), diazepam (Valium), lorazepam (Ativan), propofol (Diprivan), and dexmedetomidine (Precedex). Consider haloperidol (Haldol) if delirium present. Refer to Tab 1, Basics.
- Administer analgesics as needed. Consider morphine, fentanyl, and hydromorphone.
- Administer high doses of barbiturates to ↑ ICP and ↑ metabolic demands. Consider pentobarbital (Nembutal), phenobarbital, and thiopental (Pentothal).

- Institute seizure precautions; administer anticonvulsants as necessary. Consider phenytoin (Dilantin) (therapeutic levels 10–20 mg/mL) or carbamazepine (Tegretol). Monitor therapeutic drug levels.
- Provide DVT and stress ulcer prophylaxis.
- Prepare patient and family for possible barbiturate coma or decompression craniectomy.
- The following can ↑ ICP and should be avoided: hypercapnia, hypoxemia, Valsalva maneuver, isometric muscle contractions, REM sleep, and noxious stimuli.

Glasgow Coma Scale

Response	Patient Response	Score	Patient A	Patient B
Eye opening response	Spontaneous	4		
	To voice	3		
	To pain	2		
	None	1		
Best verbal response	Oriented	5		
	Confused	4		
	Inappropriate words	3		
	Incomprehensible sounds	2		
	None	1		
Best motor response	Obeys command	6		
	Localizes pain	5		
	Withdraws	4		
	Flexion	3		
	Extension	2		
	None	1		
Total			3–15	

A score of 8 or less indicates severe head injury.

Reprinted from Teasdale, G., and Jennett, B.: Assessment of coma and impaired consciousness: A practical scale. Lancet 304:4, 1994. Copyright 1994, with permission from Elsevier.

Full Outline of UnResponsiveness Score (FOUR Score)

Eye Response	Findings	Score
	Eyelids open and tracking, or blinking on command	4
	Eyelids open but not tracking	3

Continued

Full Outline of UnResponsiveness Score (FOUR Score)—cont'd

Eye Response	Findings	Score
	Eyelids closed but open to loud voice	2
	Eyelids closed but open to pain	1
	Eyelids closed with pain	0

Motor Response	Findings	Score
	Makes sign (thumbs-up, fist, other)	4
	Localizing to pain	3
	Flexion response to pain	2
	Extension response to pain	1
	No response to pain	0
	Generalized myoclonus status	0

Intubation	Breathing	Respiratory Score
Not intubated	Regular	4
Not intubated	Cheyne-Stokes	3
Not intubated	Irregular	2
Not intubated	Apnea	0
Intubated	Above ventilator rate	1
Intubated	Breathes at ventilator rate	0

Pupil Reflexes	Corneal Reflexes	Cough	Brainstem Score
Present	Present	Present	4
One pupil wide and fixed	Present	Present	3
Absent	Present	NA	2
Present	Absent	NA	2
Present	Absent	Absent	1
Absent	Absent	Absent	0

The total score = SUM (points for all 4 parameters). Minimum score = 0; maximum score = 16. The lower the score, the greater the coma.

From Hopkins, T.: MedSurg Notes, ed. 3. F.A. Davis, Philadelphia, 2011, pp 71–73.

Mini Mental Status Examination

Task	Instructions	Scoring	Score
Date orientation	"Tell me the date." Ask for omitted items.	1 point each for year, season, date, day of week, and month	
Place orientation	"Where are you?" Ask for omitted items.	1 point each for state, county, town, building, and floor or room.	
Register three objects	Name three objects slowly and clearly. Ask patient to repeat them.	1 point each for each item repeated correctly	
Serial 7s	Ask patient to count backward from 100 by 7. Stop after 5 answers (or ask patient to spell "world" backwards).	1 point for each correct answer (or letter)	
Recall three objects	Ask patient to recall the objects mentioned previously.	1 point for each item remembered correctly	
Naming	Point to your watch and ask, "What is this?" Repeat with a pencil.	1 point for each correct answer	
Repeating a phrase	Ask patient to say "No ifs, ands, or buts."	1 point if successful on first try	
Verbal commands	Give patient a plain piece of paper and say, "Take this paper in your right hand, fold it in half, and put it on the floor."	1 point for each correct answer	
Written commands	Show patient a piece of paper with "Close your eyes" printed on it.	1 point if patient closes eyes	

Continued

NEURO

Mini Mental Status Examination—cont'd

Task	Instructions	Scoring	Score
Writing	Ask patient to write a sentence.	1 point if sentence has a subject and a verb and makes sense	
Drawing	Ask patient to copy a pair of intersecting pentagons onto a piece of paper.	1 point if the figure has 10 corners and 2 intersecting lines	
Total possible score = 30. Score of 24 or above is considered normal.			

ICP Measurement and Monitoring
Catheters or devices placed inside the head that sense the pressure inside the brain cavity and send measurement to a recording device include:

- Intraventricular catheter (ventriculostomy), which allows CSF to drain and allows for intraventricular administration of medications
- Intraventricular fiberoptic devices
- Subarachnoid bolt or screw
- Epidural or subdural catheter or sensor/monitor

Risks
- Infection and bleeding
- Obstruction
- Damage to the brain tissue → neurological effects
- Inability to accurately place catheter

Troubleshooting ICP Monitoring Problems
- Check all connections.
- Catheter may need to be repositioned.
- Check for air in the system.
- Check monitor cable.
- Recalibrate or reposition transducer.
- Increase gain or range on monitor.
- Flush catheter with 0.25 mL NS as ordered.

ICP Catheter Waveforms
- A (plateau) waves → cerebral ischemia
- B waves → intracranial HTN and change in vascular volume
- C waves → variations in systemic arterial pressure and respirations

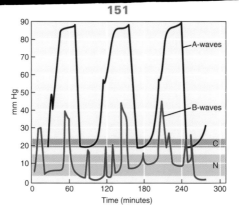

Brain Monitoring or Intraparenchymal Monitoring

Cerebral or jugular venous oxygen saturation ($SjvO_2$) (virtually all blood from the brain drains into internal jugular veins):

- 60%–80% is normal.
- <50% indicates cerebral hypoxia.
- Brain tissue O_2 monitoring (partial pressure of brain tissue O_2 [$PbtO_2$] using LICOX catheter): >25 mm Hg is normal; <20 mm Hg needs to be treated.
- Brain temperature monitoring: 0.5°C–1.0°C > core body temperature is normal.
- Bispectral index (BIS): EEG of critically ill patients with a decreased LOC is continually analyzed.

Management of CSF Drainage System

- Calibrate transducer per hospital policy. Recalibrate with any changes in patient's position. Place venting port of transducer at the level of the foramen of Monro (either tragus of ear or outer canthus of eye but must be consistent). Every 2.54 cm (1 in.) the transducer is below the pressure source → –2 mm Hg error.
- Observe ICP readings and waveforms.
- Assess neurological status and VS.
- Calculate CPP hourly; CPP = MAP – ICP.
  - Monitor and measure CSF output every hour. Note color, clarity, blood, sediment.
  - Excessive drainage may cause headache, tachycardia, nausea, or diaphoresis.

- Rapid drainage is a neurosurgical emergency.
- Stoppage of drainage may indicate a clot.
- Check dressing for drainage or signs of infection.
- Check tubing patency.
- Keep patient on bedrest with HOB 30°–45°.

Traumatic Brain Injury (TBI)

TBI refers to trauma to the scalp and skull that may or may not include injury to the brain. There are several types of acute head injuries:

- Closed head injury: The skull is not broken.
- Penetrating head injury: Object pierces the skull and breaches the dura mater.
- May also be diffuse or focal.

Pathophysiology

Trauma → intracranial hemorrhage and hematoma → brain swelling → ↑ intracranial volume and ↑ ICP → displacement or herniation of the brain. Pressure on cerebral blood vessels → ↓ blood flow to brain → ↓ O_2 to brain → cerebral hypoxia → cerebral ischemia, infarction, and irreversible brain damage → brain death.

Clinical Presentation

- Persistent, localized pain; headache
- Loss of consciousness, confusion, drowsiness, lethargy, personality change, irritability, restlessness, agitation, anterograde or retrograde amnesia
- Sudden onset of neurological deficits including hemiparesis, "doll's eyes"
- Decorticate or decerebrate posturing
- Bruising over mastoid (Battle's sign)
- Nausea and vomiting, dizziness
- CSF otorrhea (ears) or rhinorrhea (nose)
- Halo sign: blood stain surrounded by a yellowish stain on bed linens or head dressing that may indicate CSF leak
- Abnormal pupillary response; pupils may be unequal; diplopia possible
- Altered or absent gag or cough reflex
- Absent corneal reflex
- Change in vital signs: altered respiratory pattern, widened pulse pressure, bradycardia, or tachycardia; labored breathing that may be shallow and irregular with periods of apnea
- Seizures

Complicating Factors

- Skull fracture, scalp lacerations
- Cerebral contusion, concussion
- Subarachnoid hemorrhage (SAH)
- Subdural, extradural, epidural hematoma
- Cerebral edema
- ↑ ICP, ↓ cerebral perfusion, cerebral ischemia
- Seizures
- Impaired oxygenation/ventilation → respiratory depression and failure
- Infection
- Herniation, coma, persistent vegetative state, or death

Diagnostic Tests

- Check for CSF leak
- X-ray, CT of the head, MRI, or PET to assess hematoma, swelling, and injury
- TCD ultrasound
- EEG
- Cerebral angiography or CTA
- CBC, chemistry panel, and blood coagulation studies
- Global cerebral oxygenation as measured by jugular venous bulb oximetry (SjO_2). Measures mixed venous O_2 saturation of blood leaving the brain: 50%–75% normal; <50% indicates an ↑ rate O_2 extraction from cerebral ischemia
- Urinalysis for specific gravity

Management

- Management is similar to that for increased ICP.
- Stabilize cardiac and respiratory function to ensure adequate cerebral perfusion. Maintain optimum ABGs or O_2 saturation. Assess oxygenation and respiratory status. Mechanical ventilation may be needed.
- Assess and monitor neurological status and ICP; calculate CPP to maintain >70 mm Hg.
- Perform frequent neurological checks, including Glasgow Coma Scale.
- Provide light sedation as necessary to ↓ agitation. Administer analgesics for pain. Induce barbiturate coma if necessary.
- Administer hypertonic saline and osmotic diuretics (mannitol) as needed.
- Institute ICP monitoring and control for elevations in ICP.
- Induce therapeutic hypothermia.

NEURO

- Prepare patient for craniotomy or evacuation of hematoma to lessen the pressure in the brain if necessary.
- Assess for vision and hearing impairment and sensory function.
- Assess for hypothermia and hyperthermia. Control fever.
- Institute seizure precautions. Administer anticonvulsants. Minimize stimuli and excessive suctioning.
- Monitor ECG for cardiac arrhythmias.
- Institute DVT precautions.
- Assess fluid and electrolyte balance. Control hemorrhage and hypovolemia.
- Administer stool softeners to prevent Valsalva maneuver.
- Administer corticosteroids.
- Consider prophylactic antibiotics.
- Refer to Increased ICP Management for list of drugs for sedation.
- Keep head and neck in neutral alignment; no twisting or flexing of neck.
- Keep HOB elevated.
- Maintain adequate nutrition orally or enterally.
- Institute aspiration precautions as necessary.
- Assess and maintain skin integrity.
- Provide DVT and stress ulcer prophylaxis.
- Patient may be OOB when ICP controlled.

Subarachnoid Hemorrhage (SAH) or Hemorrhagic Stroke and Aneurysm Subarachnoid Hemorrhage (aSAH)

SAH is bleeding into the subarachnoid space between the arachnoid membrane and the pia mater of the brain primarily. SAH is a medical emergency.

Pathophysiology

- SAH is caused by cerebral aneurysm (usually in the area of circle of Willis), cerebral/head trauma, HTN, or arteriovenous malformation (AVM). AVM is a tangle of blood vessels without a capillary system. Aneurysms are caused by a weakening and thinning of the arterial wall → balloon or distended blood vessel and can rupture over time. Generally, aneurysms are more likely to bleed or rupture if >7 mm. Approximately 50% of aneurysms rebleed within 6 hr of initial bleeding. 25% patients have multiple aneurysms.
- Blood rapidly passes into the subarachnoid space and then spreads over the brain and to the spinal cord leading to ↑ ICP → coma → death. Bleeding can also occur intracerebrally and subdurally depending on the cause of the bleeding. Delayed cerebral ischemia can result from cerebral arterial vasospasm.

Clinical Presentation

- Sudden, severe "thunderclap" headache developing over seconds to minutes. Patient complains of it being "the worst headache in their life" (WHOL).
- Lethargy, irritability, ↓ LOC; confusion and agitation. May progress to coma.
- Pain in neck or back.
- Nuchal rigidity (stiff neck).
- Nausea and vomiting.
- Photophobia, diplopia, orbital pain, visual loss, blurred vision, and oculomotor nerve abnormalities (affected eye looking downward and outward, pupil widened and less responsive to light) involving optic, oculomotor, or trigeminal cranial nerves.
- Paralysis; positive Brudzinski's sign and Kernig's sign.
- Tinnitus, dizziness, vertigo, neurological deficits including hemiparesis.
- Fatigue, fever, and HTN.
- Cardiac arrhythmias (can progress to cardiac arrest).
- Seizures may occur early on or later.

Diagnostic Tests

- Calculate the severity of SAH using the Hunt and Hess Classification of SAH: https://www.mdcalc.com/hunt-hess-classification-subarachnoid-hemorrhage
- Hunt and Hess scale is used to classify the severity of nontraumatic SAH.

Hunt and Hess Classification of SAH	
Grade	
I	Asymptomatic, mild headache, slight nuchal rigidity
II	Moderate to severe headache, nuchal rigidity, no neurological deficit other than cranial nerve palsy
III	Drowsiness/confusion, mild focal neurological deficit
IV	Stupor, moderate to severe hemiparesis
V	Coma, decerebrate posturing

From Hunt, W.E., Hess, R.M.: Surgical risk as related to time of intervention in the repair of intracranial aneurysms. J Neurosurg 28(1):14–20, 1968.

NEURO

- Serum chemistry panel
- CBC
- PT, PTT
- Cardiac enzymes
- ABGs
- Baseline CXR
- ECG
- CT scan of brain or MRI of brain
- TCD studies
- Single photon emission computed tomography (SPECT)
- ECG (changes in ST segment and T wave, prominent U wave)
- Lumbar puncture and CSF analysis if CT inconclusive and no ↑ ICP present
- CSF clear and colorless, with no organisms present; normally tests positive for protein and glucose
- Cerebral angiography: cerebral digital subtraction angiography (DSA), multidetector computed tomography angiography (CTA)

Management

- For patients with an unavoidable delay in obliteration of aneurysm, a significant risk of rebleeding, and no compelling medical contraindications, short-term (72-hr) therapy with tranexamic acid or aminocaproic acid is reasonable to reduce the risk of early aneurysm rebleeding.
- Neurological assessment: LOC, pupillary reaction, motor and sensory function, cranial nerve deficits, and speech and visual disturbances.
- Assess for headache and nuchal rigidity.
- Provide intubation and mechanical ventilation as needed; assess ABGs and pulse oximetry.
- Monitor end-tidal CO_2, if indicated.
- Assess BP, HR, RR, and Glasgow Coma Scale frequently.
- Monitor and control fever.
- Initiate cardiac monitoring.
- Control BP with a titratable antihypertensive. Beta blockers are agents of choice in patients without contraindications. Hydralazine and Ca^{++} channel blockers have fast onset and work to lower increased ICP. Keep SBP <160 mm Hg. Balance risk or rebleeding, stroke, and CPP levels. Keep BP <160 mm Hg.
- Avoid nitrates such as NTG and vasodilators such as nitroprusside (can elevate ICP).
- Monitor and control ICP. Monitor CSF drainage systems for cloudy (infection) or bloody (rebleeding) drainage.
- Calculate and monitor CPP = MAP – ICP via ICP monitoring.
- Administer osmotic agents (mannitol), loop diuretics (Lasix).
- Consider IV steroids such as Dexamethasone (controversial).

- Monitor fluids and electrolytes.
- Insert Foley catheter if necessary and monitor urine output.
- Consider packed RBC transfusions to treat anemia.
- Monitor and control blood glucose levels.
- Institute seizure precautions and start antiepileptic drug (AED) therapy.
- Institute aneurysm precautions: bedrest; dark, quiet room with minimal stimulation and nonstressful environment; pain control (consider fentanyl); ↑ HOB 15°–30°; stool softeners and bowel regimen (avoid enemas). Restrict visitors.
- Avoid Valsalva maneuver, straining, forceful sneezing, and acute flexion of head and neck. Eliminate caffeine from diet.
- Administer analgesics for pain control; use nonsedating agents. Control anxiety. Consider midazolam.
- Administer nimodipine (Nymalize) for cerebral vasodilation. Therapy should start within 96 hr of SAH.
- Provide DVT and stress ulcer prophylaxis.
- Monitor and treat heparin-induced thrombocytopenia.

Triple-H Therapy to Prevent Vasospasms

- Hypovolemia is treated with colloids and crystalloids to keep CVP 10–12 mm Hg and PCWP 14–20 mm Hg.
- Hemodilution is used to keep hematocrit level at 33%–38%.
- Hypertensive therapy is given to keep SBP 110–160 mm Hg.
- Also monitor levels of oxygenation.
- Administer oral nimodipine.
  Prepare patient for surgery:
- Surgical aneurysm repair: surgical clipping. Complete obliteration of aneurysm recommended.
- Endovascular (aneurysm) coiling: obstruction of aneurysm site with coil. Coiling preferred over clipping.
- After aneurysm repair, immediate cerebrovascular imaging is recommended to identify remnants or recurrence of aneurysm.
- Stenting of a ruptured aneurysm is not recommended.

Complications

Additional management is aimed at preventing the following complications:

- Increased ICP
- Coma and brainstem herniation
- Rebleeding: greatest risk within first 24 hr of rupture. Assess for ↑ ICP and fresh bloody CSF, sudden and severe headache, altered LOC, new neurological deficits
- Cerebral vasospasm, delayed cerebral ischemia, cerebral infarction, changes in LOC, headache, new neurological deficits, seizures

NEURO

- Seizures
- Hyponatremia from SIADH or cerebral salt-wasting syndrome
- Heparin-induced thrombocytopenia
- Cardiac arrhythmias and myocardial damage
- Acute hydrocephalus: managed by external ventricular drainage or lumbar drainage
- Pneumonia, DVT, pulmonary embolus, and respiratory failure
- Neurogenic cardiac stunning (reduction of function of heart contraction) and pulmonary edema

Management of Cerebral Vasospasm and Delayed Cerebral Ischemia After aSAH

- Oral nimodipine should be administered to all patients with aSAH. (This agent has been shown to improve neurological outcomes but not cerebral vasospasm. The value of other calcium antagonists, oral or IV, remains uncertain.)
- Maintenance of euvolemia and normal circulating blood volume is recommended to prevent delayed cerebral ischemia.
- Prophylactic hypervolemia or balloon angioplasty before the development of angiographic spasm is not recommended.
- TCD is reasonable to monitor for the development of arterial vasospasm.
- Perfusion imaging with CT or MRI can be useful to identify regions of potential brain ischemia.
- Induction of HTN is recommended for patients with delayed cerebral ischemia unless BP is elevated at baseline or cardiac status precludes it. Cerebral angioplasty or selective intra-arterial vasodilator therapy is reasonable in patients with symptomatic cerebral vasospasm, particularly those who are not rapidly responding to hypertensive therapy.

Cerebral Vascular Accident (CVA): Ischemic Stroke

CVA is a sudden disruption of blood flow to a part of the brain resulting in brain tissue damage and neurological deficits. CVA is also called brain attack or stroke.

Pathophysiology

- Causes of CVA include thrombosis, embolism, systemic hypoperfusion. Cocaine use doubles the risk of CVA.

- In CVA, disruption of blood flow to the brain → ↓ O_2 and glucose to the brain → ischemic cascade → neurons unable to maintain aerobic respiration → switch to anaerobic respiration → buildup of lactic acid → change in blood pH → influx of intracellular calcium and increase in glutamate → destroys cell membrane → cell membrane and proteins break down, forming free radicals → cell injury and death → neurological dysfunction.
- Low cerebral blood flow → ↓ O_2 to the brain → ↑ extraction of O_2 by the brain.
- Ischemia penumbra (zone of ischemic area) forms around an infarct in stroke lesions. This penumbra may be reversible.

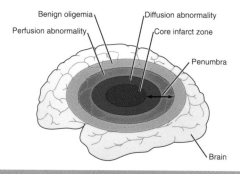

Benign oligemia · Diffusion abnormality · Perfusion abnormality · Core infarct zone · Penumbra · Brain

Clinical Presentation

- Sudden neurological deficits such as muscle weakness (hemiplegia) of face, arm, or leg (especially if confined to one side of body); confusion or trouble speaking or understanding speech; trouble seeing in one or both eyes; trouble walking; dizziness; loss of balance or coordination; and severe headache with no known cause
- Other neurological assessments: sudden ↓ LOC, ptosis (drooping of eyelids), weakness of ocular muscles, ↓ gag and swallow reflex, slow papillary reactivity to light, visual field defects, memory defects, confusion, and hypersexual gestures
- Numbness; ↓ sensory or vibratory sensation; altered sense of smell, taste, hearing; ↓ sensation and muscle weakness to face (facial paresis); nystagmus; and dysphagia
- Altered breathing and heart rate

NEURO

- Inability to turn head to one side (weak sternocleidomastoid muscle)
- Inability to protrude tongue and/or move it from side to side
- Aphasia (difficult to speak or understand language)
- Apraxia (altered voluntary movements)
- Vertigo and disequilibrium, with difficulty walking, altered movement coordination, and arm drift
- Urinary and fecal incontinence

Complications

- Physical: pressure sores, incontinence, pneumonia, seizures, coma, and death
- Emotional: anxiety, panic attacks, flat affect, depression, withdrawal, sleep disturbances, lethargy, irritability, and emotional lability

Diagnostic Tests

- The timing and use of diagnostics highly depends on the time of admission and on whether the patient is a candidate for rtPA or is post-procedure rtPA
- Calculate NIH Stroke Score for quantifying stroke severity:
  - http://reference.medscape.com/calculator/nih-stroke-score
  - http://www.mdcalc.com/nih-stroke-scale-score-nihss/
- CBC with platelet count
- Serum chemistry including electrolytes, glucose and renal function tests; consider hepatic function tests
- Coagulation studies
- Cardiac biomarkers, especially troponin
- Toxicology screen and blood ETOH level if indicated because stroke symptoms may mimic substance abuse
- Pregnancy testing
- Noncontrast brain CT or brain MRI
- CXR if lung disease suspected
- CT/MRI perfusion and diffusion imaging
- Carotid artery vascular ultrasound or carotid Doppler ultrasound
- ECG, especially if atrial fibrillation suspected
- Consider EEG, especially if seizure activity present; consider lumbar puncture if SAH or CNS infection suspected
- O₂ saturation and ABGs if suspected hypoxia
- Vascular imaging: CTA; intracranial MRA, TCD ultrasonography, DSA, conventional angiography

Management

Based on the American Heart Association/American Stroke Association Guidelines for the Early Management of Patients with Acute Ischemic Stroke (https://www.ahajournals.org/doi/abs/10.1161/str.0000000000000158):

- ■ Administer recombinant tissue plasminogen activator (rtPA) within 3–4.5 hr of onset of symptoms if eligibility criteria are met.
- ■ Alteplase is recommended. Streptokinase is not recommended.
- ■ The greatest benefits are seen in patients treated within 90 min of symptom onset.
- ■ Door to needle time within 60 min of hospital arrival if patient eligible for IV fibrinolysis.
- ■ Antiplatelet agents and anticoagulants are contraindicated during the first 24 hr after IV rtPA treatment.
- ■ Administer 325 mg aspirin within 24–48 hr after stroke onset.
- ■ Use of clopidogrel (Plavix), tirofiban (Aggrastat), and eptifibatide (Integrilin) is not well established.
- ■ Use of argatroban (Acova, Novastan) is not well established.
- ■ Initiation of anticoagulant therapy within 24 hr of treatment with intravenous rtPA is not recommended.
- ■ Assess for bleeding related to therapy, including intracranial hemorrhage.
- ■ Use of induced hypothermia is not well established. Consider use in select patients.
- ■ Assess and monitor neurological status for increasing neurological deficits.
- ■ Assess and monitor respiratory function because hypoxia frequently occurs. Administer O_2 only as necessary by cannula, mask, BiPAP, or CPAP, or intubate and place on mechanical ventilation as needed. Keep O_2 saturation at >94%.
- ■ Monitor and manage ↑ ICP and cerebral edema. Administer mannitol or furosemide (Lasix). Corticosteroids are not recommended.
- ■ Administer IV fluids cautiously in patients with cardiac or renal disease. Correct hypovolemia with IV 0.9% normal saline. Avoid IV dextrose solutions, 0.45% NS, and albumin.
- ■ Monitor and control BP cautiously. Initially lower SBP by 15% while monitoring for neurological worsening. BP must be <185/100 mm Hg before IV rtPA. After rtPA, maintain BP <185/110 mm Hg for at least 24 hr after starting therapy. Administer labetalol 10–20 mg IV over 1–2 min, repeat 1 time; or nicardipine 5 mg/hr IV, titrate up by 2.5 mg/hr every 5–15 min, maximum 15 mg/hr. Consider hydralazine and enalapril. If BP not controlled or DBP >140 mm Hg, consider IV nitroprusside. Vasodilators not recommended. Use vasopressors if patient is hypotensive.
- ■ Provide DVT and stress ulcer disease prophylaxis if patient is immobilized.

- Maintain glycemic control. Administer IV insulin cautiously to prevent hypoglycemia. Target serum glucose levels <60 and <140–180 mg/dL.
- Provide either continuous ECG monitoring or Holter monitoring to detect bradycardia ← ↓ cardiac output and ↑ CPP and arrhythmias especially atrial fibrillation.
- Treat and control fever. Administer antibiotics for pneumonia and UTIs. Prophylactic antibiotics not recommended.
- Avoid use of Foley catheter if possible. Monitor intake and output closely.
- Institute seizure precautions, and administer anticonvulsants if necessary.
- Provide enteral or PEG tube feedings, following aspiration precautions.
- Elevate HOB 30°. Consider swallowing assessment.

Endovascular Interventions

- Intra-arterial fibrinolysis
- A combination of IV and intra-arterial fibrinolysis
- Mechanical thrombectomy to remove offending thrombus with select thrombus retrievers
- Extra-intracranial bypass (EC-IC) not recommended; no benefit shown over medical therapy
- Use of intracranial angioplasty and/or stenting not well established

Herniation of the Brain

A brain herniation occurs when brain tissue, CSF, and blood vessels are moved away from their usual position inside the skull. May result from brain swelling caused by a head injury, stroke, or brain tumor. Other causes include abscess, hemorrhage, hydrocephalus, and swelling after radiation therapy. Brain herniation can cause a massive stroke and can quickly lead to brain death or death.

Signs and symptoms:

- Cardiac arrest
- Cushing's triad of impending herniation: an increase in pulse pressure; bradycardia; and slow, irregular respiratory rate
- Headache
- Lethargy, difficulty concentrating, drowsy or agitated ← stupor and coma
- Loss of brainstem reflexes such as blinking, gagging
- Changes in pupillary reaction, sluggish ← fixed and dilated pupils
- Hemiparesis ← decortication, decerebration, flaccidity
- Increased BP, irregular and slow HR
- Increased BP, hyperventilation ← irregular breathing ← Cheyne-Stokes ← respiratory arrest

Management

- Brain herniation is a medical emergency.
- Refer to ICP section.
- Insert catheter to remove CSF.
- Administer corticosteroids (dexamethasone).
- Administer mannitol.
- Intubate and put patient on mechanical ventilation to reduce CO_2 levels.
- Remove blood or blood clots if causing herniation.
- Remove part of the skull.

Spinal Cord Injury (SCI)

SCI may be classified as complete (loss of conscious sensory and motor function below the level of SCI as a result of transection of the spinal cord) or incomplete (preservation of some sensory and motor function below the level of SCI as a result of partial spinal cord transection). The most common sites of SCI are C4–C7, T12, and L1.

Causes of SCI include:

- Motor vehicle accidents
- Diving accidents
- Falls
- Blunt force trauma
- Penetrating force trauma
- Spinal abscesses and tumors, especially lymphoma and multiple myeloma

Pathophysiology

- ↓ blood flow to gray matter of spinal cord with 8-hr delay of ↓ blood flow to white matter → thrombi form furthering ↓ blood flow to spinal cord.
- ↑ interstitial pressure related to edema → ↓ blood flow to spinal cord.
- Inflammatory process → edema of injured area → ↓ blood flow to spinal cord. Edema moves up and down the spinal cord rather than laterally.
- Release of norepinephrine, histamine, and prostaglandins → vasoconstriction → ↓ cellular perfusion.
- ↑ extracellular fluid concentrations of Na^+ and K^+ → ↑ osmotic pressure in area of injury → edema.
- Ischemia, hypoxia, and edema → tissue necrosis and cell membrane damage → destruction of myelin and axons → neuronal death.

NEURO

Clinical Presentation

- Spinal shock initially: flaccid paralysis with ↑ or absent reflex activity
- Partial or total loss of motor function below the level of SCI (includes voluntary movement and movement against gravity or resistance)
- Partial or total loss of sensory function below the level of SCI (includes touch, temperature, pain, proprioception [e.g., position])
- ↑ HR initially → bradycardia; ↑ BP initially ↑ → ↓ BP
- Acute pain in back or neck that may radiate along nerve
- Abnormal deep tendon reflex and perianal reflex activity
- Loss of sweating and vagomotor tone
- Loss of sensory, motor, and deep tendon reflexes below the level of injury
- Retention of lung secretions, ↑ vital capacity, ↑ Paco₂, ↑ O₂ → respiratory failure and pulmonary edema
- Bladder and bowel incontinence with urine retention and bladder distention
- Paralytic ileus causing constipation and/or bowel impaction
- Loss of temperature control → hyperthermia
- Sweating above level of lesion
- Priapism in male patients
- Associated injuries resulting from trauma: broken teeth, swollen tongue, neurological and orthopedic injuries, hemothorax, pneumothorax, flail chest, intrathoracic injuries, abdominal and retroperitoneal injuries

Diagnostic Tests

- Lateral, anteroposterior (cervical, thoracic, lumbar, sacral), and odontoid films
- CXR and ECG
- CT scan, MRI
- Myelography
- Standard Neurological Classification of Spinal Cord Injury categorizes motor and sensory impairments in SCI indicating the lowest spinal levels demonstrating "unimpaired function." The following worksheet may be downloaded at: http://www.asia-spinalinjury.org/elearning/ ISNCSCI_Exam_Sheet_r4.pdf
- American Spinal Injury Association (ASIA) Impairment Scale
  - A = Complete: No motor or sensory function is preserved in the sacral segments S4–S5.
  - B = Incomplete: Sensory but no motor function is preserved below the neurological level and includes the sacral segments S4–S5.
  - C = Incomplete: Motor function is preserved below the neurological level, and more than half of key muscles below the neurological level have a muscle grade less than 3.

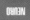

- D = Incomplete: Motor function is preserved below the neurological level, and at least half of key muscles below the neurological level have a muscle grade of 3 or more.
- E = Normal: Motor and sensory function are normal.

Note: Loss of motor function means a person has no voluntary control of his or her muscles. Loss of sensory function means a person has no sense of touch and cannot feel hot or cold, pain, or pressure. The person also has no sense of where in space his or her limbs are.

- Routine blood tests: CBC, serum chemistry panel, toxicology if suspected ETOH or substance abuse, coagulation studies, ABGs, lactate, urinalysis

Management

- Stabilize and support the spine through various devices and specialized beds/frames.
- Assess motor and sensory function, including deep tendon reflexes.
- Assess neurological status, including LOC and papillary action.
- Assess for closed head injury.
- Maintain spinal and proper body alignment.
- Assess respiratory status. Monitor ABGs or pulse oximetry. Administer O_2 by nasal cannula or mask. Provide mechanical ventilation as determined by ABGs.
- Monitor pulmonary function: tidal volume, minute volume, inspiratory force.
- Suction cautiously → stimulate vagus nerve → bradycardia → cardiac arrest.
- Monitor ECG for cardiac dysrhythmias, especially bradycardia (may need atropine or pacemaker). Monitor BP for hypotension. Administer vasopressors (dopamine, dobutamine, phenylephrine) as needed.
- Provide intermittent bladder catheterization or temporary Foley catheter.
- Provide DVT and stress ulcer prophylaxis.
- Insert nasogastric tube initially to prevent vomiting and aspiration.
- Assess bowel sounds and abdomen for paralytic ileus and/or distention.
- Stabilize body temperature resulting from problems with thermoregulation.
- Administer analgesics as necessary.
- Control skeletal muscle spasms by administering dantrolene (Dantrium), baclofen (Lioresal), or tizanidine (Zanaflex).
- Start oral or enteral feedings. Consider TPN as necessary.
- Institute safety precautions.
- Follow skin care protocol to prevent pressure ulcers.
- Insert Foley catheter as necessary and monitor urine output. Avoid and treat bladder spasms.

NEURO

- Avoid bowel impaction by administering stool softeners and establish bowel control.
- Prevent autonomic dysreflexia.
- Provide IV fluids cautiously because they can precipitate heart failure as a result of poor heart rate response to ↑ circulating blood volume.
- Administer crystalloids and blood products as indicated.
- Administration of methylprednisolone Na succinate within 8 hr of injury (30 mg/kg IV over 15 min; infusion of 5.4 mg/kg/hr for 24–48 hr) remains controversial and is associated with severe pneumonia and sepsis.
- Administer vasodilators as needed: nitroglycerine, nifedipine (Procardia), phenoxybenzamine (Dibenzyline), hydralazine or nitroprusside (Nipride).
- Prevent sepsis and infections (respiratory, urinary tract, and wound).
- Provide emotional support for patient and family.
- Prepare patient for surgical management to reduce spinal fracture or dislocation and decompression of the spinal cord:
  - Skeletal fracture reduction and traction with skeletal tongs or calipers, skeletal traction device, and halo device

Autonomic Dysreflexia

Autonomic dysreflexia is also known as hyperreflexia. It occurs in people with SCI at or above the level of T5–T7 and rarely as low as T8. It is considered a medical emergency because it precipitates life-threatening HTN.

A stimulus causes ↑ sympathetic nervous system response below the level of SCI and systemic vasoconstriction of blood vessels → bradycardia, sudden ↑ in SBP and DBP, facial and neck flushing (reddening above the level of SCI) associated with pale, cold skin on the trunk and extremities (below the SCI), sweating, anxiety, pounding headache, nausea, metallic taste, nasal congestion, "goose bumps," blurred vision, difficulty breathing, increased spasticity, and chest pain. It may lead to CVA, renal failure, atrial fibrillation, seizures, and acute pulmonary edema.

Causes

- Numerous causes including fractures, surgery, diagnostic procedures, and a variety of medical conditions
- Bladder distention or spasm (most common cause): UTI
- Bowel distention or impaction
- Stimulation of anal reflex (stimulation of skin around the anus produces contraction of the anal sphincter)
- Gastric irritation including gastric ulcers or gastritis
- Menstruation, vaginitis, sexual intercourse, ejaculation
- Labor and delivery in women

- Temperature change
- Acute pain
- Spasticity
- DVT and pulmonary embolus
- Pressure ulcers
- Burns, blisters, sunburn, insect bites
- Tight, constrictive clothes or shoes
- Ingrown toenails

Management

- Place patient in sitting position and monitor vital signs every 5 min.
- Loosen constrictive clothing or devices.
- If no indwelling catheter, palpate bladder for distention → insert Foley catheter.
- If indwelling catheter, check for kinks and obstruction and irrigate if necessary.
- Check for fecal impaction and administer laxative as needed. Use 2% lidocaine jelly 10–15 min before removing impaction.
- Assess skin for pressure or irritation.
- If SBP >150 mm Hg, administer an antihypertensive such as nifedipine (Procardia) sublingually and nitrates (nitroglycerine paste) as first line of treatment. Consider hydralazine (Apresoline), mecamylamine (less commonly used), phenoxybenzamine (Dibenzyline), diazoxide (Hyperstat).
  - The sweating will become less profuse or stop.
  - There will usually be an immediate lowering of the BP, although it may take about 1 hr for BP to decrease if BP is very high.
- Fatal complications include pneumonia, renal failure, pulmonary embolism, and septicemia.

Neurogenic Shock

Neurogenic shock generally occurs in SCIs above T6. It may develop in days or months after the injury.

Neurogenic shock is caused by vasoconstriction and venous pooling (veins dilated and filled with blood) → ↓ BP, ↓ systemic vascular resistance, ↓ HR, ↓ CO, ↓ respiration rate → ↓ blood flow to vital organs → organ damage and ischemia. The patient may also have the inability to sweat below the level of injury → hypothermia.

Treatment involves the administration of vasopressors, atropine, and treatment of hypothermia.

NEURO

Myasthenia Gravis (MG)

MG is a neuromuscular autoimmune disease causing muscle weakness and fatigability of skeletal muscles.

Pathophysiology

Circulating antibodies block acetylcholine receptors at the postsynaptic neuro-muscular junction → inhibits acetylcholine → inhibits depolarization of muscles → ↓ nerve impulse transmission → diminishes muscle contraction, including diaphragmatic muscle → ↓ vital capacity and respiratory failure.
Causes include thymic hyperplasia and tumor of the thymus gland.

Clinical Presentation

- Abnormal muscle weakness that increases during activity and improves after rest; eye muscle weakness; possible ptosis, diplopia, and inability to maintain upward gaze
- Weakness of limb, axial, bulbar, and/or respiratory muscles, especially those related to chewing, talking, swallowing (dysphagia), breathing, and neck and limb movements; inability to close mouth and inability to raise chin off chest
- Slurred speech, neck muscle weakness with head bobbing
- Diaphragmatic and intercostal weakness → dyspnea, difficulty coughing
- Crises that may be triggered by fever, infection, trauma, extreme temperatures, adverse reaction to medication or emotional stress → respiratory distress, dysphagia, dysarthria (difficulty speaking), eyelid ptosis, diplopia, prominent muscle weakness, neurological changes, absence of sweating, hyperthermia → respiratory failure
- Myasthenia crisis manifested by respiratory paralysis

Diagnostic Tests

- Muscle fatigability test
- Antibodies against acetylcholine receptor (AChR Abs) ≤0.03 nmol/L or negative
- Edrophonium chloride (Tension) test: Available as 10 mg/mL. Administer 2 mg IV over 15-20 sec; resolution of facial muscle weakness and ptosis and improved muscle strength should be seen in 30 sec; if no response in 45 sec, inject the remaining 8 mg. May repeat the test after 30 min; have atropine, ECG monitoring, and advanced life-saving equipment available

- Ice pack test: Placing ice over an eyelid if ptosis is present; clear resolution of the ptosis is a positive test result; ptosis occurs in approximately 80% of patients with ocular myasthenia
- Single-fiber electromyography and repetitive nerve stimulation
- Blood test to identify antibodies against the acetylcholine receptor (AChR Abs)
- Thyroid function and PFTs
- CXR, CT scan, or MRI to detect thymomas

Management

- Assess and monitor respiratory status and oxygenation (PFTs, ABGs).
- Provide mechanical ventilation if paralysis of respiratory muscles is present. Consider NIPPV.
- Monitor for and treat bronchospasm: albuterol (Proventil, Ventolin), ipratropium (Atrovent), glycopyrrolate (Robinul).
- Monitor risk for aspiration and pneumonia. Initiate enteral feedings if dysphagic.
- Avoid sedatives and tranquilizers.
- Initiate plasmapheresis to treat exacerbations.
- Administer intervenous immune globulin (IVIG).
- Administer corticosteroids: prednisone, methylprednisolone (Solu-Medrol).
- Administer immunomodulators: azathioprine (Imuran, Azasan), cyclosporine (Neoral, Sandimmune), cyclophosphamide, mycophenolate mofetil (CellCept), rituximab (Rituxan), tacrolimus (Prograf).
- Administer acetylcholine esterase (AChE) inhibitors: neostigmine (Prostigmin), pyridostigmine (Mestinon).
- Provide DVT and stress ulcer prophylaxis.
- Prepare patient for surgical thymectomy.

Guillain-Barré Syndrome (GBS)

GBS is an autoimmune acute inflammatory disease causing demyelination of the lower motor neurons of the peripheral nervous system. It is also sometimes referred to as acute idiopathic polyneuritis of infectious polyneuritis.

Pathophysiology

- Immune-mediated response → destruction of myelin sheath → interferes with nerve signal transmission → slowing of nerve signals → weakness of limbs → ascending paralysis → total paralysis.
- Paralysis of the diaphragm → respiratory failure and respiratory arrest.
- If mild, remyelination can occur.

Clinical Presentation

- Infection of the respiratory or GI tract 7–14 days before onset of neurological symptoms
- Symmetrical muscle weakness → flaccidity of muscle → symmetrical ascending paralysis from the legs (hours or days) leading to upper limbs and face with/without numbness or tingling
- Loss of deep tendon reflexes (areflexia)
- Difficulty with eye movements; double vision
- Difficulty with swallowing; drooling; facial droop
- Loss of pain and temperature sensation
- Loss of proprioception (position sense)
- Sinus tachycardia or bradycardia and cardiac dysrhythmias
- Orthostatic hypotension; HTN
- Absence of fever; excessive diaphoresis
- Urinary retention common leading to UTI
- Seizures
- Bowel and bladder retention or incontinence
- Decrease in vital capacity and negative inspiratory force → respiratory failure/arrest
- ↑ pulmonary secretions
- SIADH
- ↓ protein in CSF (100–1,000 mg/dL)
- Residual damage possibly occurring after the acute phase

Diagnostic Tests

- Lumbar puncture and CSF analysis
- EMG and nerve conduction velocity studies
- CBC, PFTs, and ABGs
- Serum immunoglobulin

Management

- Assess respiratory status and ABGs.
- Provide early respiratory support, including mechanical ventilation with or without tracheostomy.
- Assess neurological function especially sensory and motor loss; start with lower extremities. Assess LOC.
- ECG and BP monitoring. Treat dysrhythmias.
- Administer antihypertensive or vasopressors to maintain BP within normal limits. Consider IV fluid resuscitation as indicated.

- Monitor for and provide preventive care for infections caused by complications: pneumonia, UTIs, septicemia.
- Insert indwelling Foley catheter if appropriate.
- Provide enteral feedings and nutritional support.
- Active and passive range of motion and physical or occupational therapy are provided.
- Corticosteroids such as prednisone may be tried but generally are not effective.
- Administer IVIG at 400 mg/kg for 5 consecutive days.
- Plasmapheresis (therapeutic plasma exchange): two sessions for patients with mild disease, 4 exchanges for moderate disease, up to 6 exchanges for severe disease. Side effects increase with number of exchanges.
- Provide DVT and stress ulcer prophylaxis.
- Institute safety precautions if changes in mental status occur.
- Provide short- and long-term rehabilitation, physical therapy, and occupational therapy consultations.
- Complications include:
  - Loss of bowel and bladder control
  - Pressure ulcers, contractures and muscle wasting
  - Thrombophlebitis
  - Respiratory tract infections, respiratory failure and sepsis

Bacterial Meningitis

Bacterial meningitis is an inflammation that involves the arachnoid and pia mater of the brain, the subarachnoid space, and the CSF.

Pathophysiology

- Bacteria enter the CNS through the bloodstream and cross the blood-brain barrier or directly enter the bloodstream via penetrating trauma, invasive procedures, cancer, certain drugs, or ruptured cerebral abscess. An upper respiratory infection → bacteria in nasopharynx → bloodstream → CSF subarachnoid space and pia-arachnoid membrane → meninges.
- Purulent exudate → clings to meningeal layers → clogs CSF → tissue and vascular congestion and obstruction → cranial nerve dysfunction, hyperemia of meningeal blood vessels, brain tissue edema, ↑ CSF, ↑ ICP, ↑ WBC in subarachnoid space → acute hydrocephalus and seizures.
- Abnormal stimulation of hypothalamic area → inappropriate ADH production → water retention.

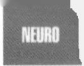

Clinical Presentation

- Symptoms of upper respiratory infection possibly preceding meningeal irritation → severe and unrelenting headache, nausea, vomiting, fever and chills, nuchal rigidity (stiff neck), irritability, malaise, restlessness, myalgia, and tachycardia
- Photophobia and signs of ↑ ICP
- Problems with memory; ↓ LOC; disorientation to person, place, and year; sleepiness, confusion, irritability, abnormal eye movements → coma, delirium, and seizures
- Kernig's sign: inability to extend the leg at the knee when the thigh is flexed
- Brudzinski's sign: flexion of the hip and knee when the patient's neck is flexed

Complications

- Septic emboli and septic shock with vascular dysfunction, or DIC
- Pericardial effusion
- Fluid and electrolyte imbalances
- Seizures and hemiparesis
- Cranial nerve (CN) dysfunction: CN III, IV, VI, VII, VIII
- Cerebral infarction, brain parenchymal damage
- Hydrocephalus and cerebral edema
- ↑ ICP → herniation of the brain

Diagnostic Tests

- Lumbar puncture, culture, and assessment of CSF and pressure → ↑ CSF pressure (CSF pressure >180 mm Hg is indicative of bacterial meningitis); CSF fluid cloudy with ↑ protein, ↓ glucose, ↑ WBCs and neutrophils
- CBC, especially ↑ WBC
- PT/INR/PTT
- Blood cultures and cultures from nasopharynx, respiratory secretions, urine
- Serum electrolytes, especially Na (dilutional hyponatremia), BUN, glucose
- CXR to determine concomitant pneumonia
- CT scan or MRI if ↑ ICP, or brain abscess or hydrocephalus

Management

Infectious Diseases Society of America Guidelines on Diagnosis of Healthcare-Associated Ventriculitis and Meningitis: https://emedicine.staging.medscape.com/article/232915-guidelines

- Maintain respiratory isolation until pathogen is not cultured in nasopharynx (usually 24 hr after antibiotic treatment).
- Monitor neurological status, cranial nerve function, and vital signs every 1–2 hr. Check pupils, LOC, and motor activity.
- Assess vascular function for signs of septic emboli.
- Ensure ↓ environmental stimuli, quiet environment, and ↓ exposure to lights.
- Administer corticosteroids to decrease inflammation: dexamethasone.
- Administer anticonvulsants for seizures: phenytoin, phenobarbital, lorazepam.
- Administer antipyretics for fever.
- Administer analgesia for headache.
- Administer hyperosmolar agents for cerebral edema: mannitol and diuretics: Lasix.
- Insert surgical shunt if hydrocephalus is present and adjust antibiotic therapy per the causative agent and antibiotic sensitivity.
- Consider the following antibiotic therapy:
    - Cefotaxime (Claforan)
    - Ceftazidime (Ceptaz, Fortaz)
    - Ceftriaxone (Rocephin)
    - Vancomycin
    - Meropenem (Merrem)

Assess CSF analysis, Gram stain, and cultures for antibiotic sensitivity.

Seizure Disorder

A seizure disorder is a temporary, abnormal, sudden, excessive, uncontrolled electrical discharge of neurons of the cerebral cortex. Status epilepticus (SE), which denotes continuous seizure activity (lasting >5 min or two or more sequential seizures), is a medical emergency.

Pathophysiology

Repetitive depolarization of hyperactive hypersensitive brain cells → abnormal electrical activity in the brain.

Risk factors for seizure disorder include:

- Epilepsy
- Drug or alcohol abuse
- Drug toxicity (aminophylline)
- Recent head injury
- Infection
- Headache

- Acute metabolic disturbances (hypoglycemia, hyponatremia, hypocalcemia, renal failure)
- CVA
- CNS infection (meningitis, encephalitis)
- CNS trauma or tumor
- Hypoxemia
- Fever (children)
- HTN
- Allergic reaction
- Eclampsia related to pregnancy

Clinical Presentation

- From simple staring to prolonged convulsions
- Brief loss of memory, sparkling or flashes, and sensing of an unpleasant odor
- Classified as motor, sensory, autonomic, emotional, or cognitive
- Aura occurring before the seizure, along with tachycardia
- Alteration in mental state; confusion or dazed state
- Automatisms such as lip smacking or chewing
- Tonic or clonic movements
- Loss of consciousness or inability to respond to external stimuli
- No memory of recent events
- Déjà vu or jamais vu (any familiar situation that is not recognized by the observer)

The clinical presentation of seizure disorder depends on the type of seizure.

Complications

- Pulmonary edema
- Pulmonary aspiration
- Cardiac dysrhythmias
- HTN or hypotension
- Hyperthermia
- Hyperglycemia/hypoglycemia
- Hypoxia
- Dehydration and metabolic imbalances
- Myoglobinuria
- Oral or musculoskeletal injuries
- Brain death

Diagnostic Tests

- EEG
- CT scan, MRI, or PET to rule out cerebral lesions
- Serum drug screen to rule out drug or alcohol intoxication
- Serum electrolytes, BUN, calcium, magnesium, glucose
- CBC
- ECG to detect cardiac arrhythmias
- ABGs or pulse oximetry

Management

- The primary aim of seizure management is to protect the airway and prevent injury to the patient. Refer to Guidelines for the Evaluation and Management of Status Epilepticus (2012): neurocriticalcare.ucsd.edu/wp -content/.../NCS-StausEpilepticus-Guideline-2012.pdf
- Administer fast-acting anticonvulsants:
  - Lorazepam (Ativan): 0.1 mg/kg up to 4 mg per dose IV. Administer no faster than 2 mg/min. May repeat in 5–10 min. Treatment of choice.
  - Midazolam: 0.2 mg/kg IM up to 10 mg maximum.
  - Diazepam (Valium): 0.15 mg/kg IV up to 10 mg per dose. Administer no faster than 5 mg/min. May repeat in 5 min.
- Administer long-acting anticonvulsants:
  - Phenytoin (Dilantin): 20 mg/kg IV. Administer no faster than 50 mg/min. May give an additional 5–10 mg/kg 10 min after loading infusion.
  - Phenobarbital (Luminal): 20 mg/kg IV. Administer no faster than 50–100 mg/min. May give an additional 5–10 mg/kg 10 min after loading infusion.
  - Fosphenytoin (Cerebyx): 20 mg/kg IV. Administer no faster than 150 mg/min. May give an additional 5 mg/kg 10 min after loading infusion.
  - Propofol (Diprivan): dosage per anesthesiologist.
  - Midazolam (Versed): dosage per anesthesiologist.
- Other anticonvulsants for seizure control maintenance are given orally and are not for acute seizure activity:
  - Carbamazepine (Tegretol)
  - Gabapentin (Neurontin)
  - Levetiracetam (Keppra)
  - Valproate (Depakote)
- Identify precipitating factors and preceding aura.
  - What was the patient doing at the time of the seizure?
  - Were there any unusual symptoms or behaviors before the seizure (e.g., movements, sensations, sounds, tastes, smells)?
  - Did the patient know he or she was going to have a seizure?

NEURO

During seizure:

- Observe seizure type, point of origin, and spread of seizure activity.
- Note length of time of the seizure.
- Note automatisms, such as lip smacking and repeated biting.
- Assess LOC, bowel and bladder incontinence, and tongue biting.
- Avoid restraining the patient.
- Avoid forcing airway into patient's mouth when jaws clenched.
- Avoid use of tongue blade.
- Maintain patent airway during seizure.
- During postictal state (after seizure):
- Assess vital signs closely; provide ECG monitoring.
- Monitor oxygenation and respiratory status (ABGs, SpO_2, breath sounds).
- Turn patient to side-lying position; administer O_2 therapy; suction prn.
- Check level of orientation and ability to speak (patient usually sleeps afterward).
- Note headache and signs of increased ICP.
- Check pupil size, eye deviations, and response to auditory and tactile stimuli.
- Note paralysis or weakness of arms or legs.
- Keep oral or nasal airway or ETT at bedside.
- Ensure patient's safety (pad side rails, bed at lowest position).
- Prevent Wernicke-Korsakoff syndrome; administer thiamine 100 mg IV and 50 mL of 50% glucose if chronic alcohol ingestion or hypoglycemia is present.
- Surgery may be indicated in select cases.

Neurosurgery

Indications include tumors, AVMs and aneurysms. Craniotomy is the most common procedure. Others include stereotactic biopsy and neuroendoscopy.

Complications

- Neurological deficits: some may be expected, others not
- Cerebral edema, increased ICP, hydrocephalus, CSF leak
- Vasogenic edema
- Cerebral infarction
- Seizures
- Pneumocephalus
- Infections: wound, meningitis, abscesses
- Hemorrhage
- Hyponatremia and electrolyte imbalances such as SIADH, cerebral salt wasting
- DVT and pulmonary embolism

Postoperative Care

- Provide routine critical care post-op nursing interventions with focus on neurological assessment and CSF leakage, especially from the ear, nose, and surgical site.
- Control BP.
- Consider corticosteroids and osmotic diuretics.
- Administer anticonvulsants.
- Perform DVT and stress ulcer prophylaxis.
- Avoid excessive suction with drainage devices.
- Note a swallow evaluation may be indicated before starting oral fluids.
- Avoid IV fluids with dextrose. Use hypertonic solutions.

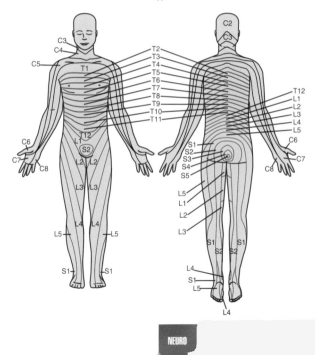

61

Acute Gastrointestinal Bleeding

Causes of upper GI (UGI) bleeding include:

- Gastric or duodenal ulcers including stress-related ulceration; nonsteroidal anti-inflammatory drugs (NSAIDs)–related peptic ulcer disease, erosive or hemorrhagic gastritis, or esophagitis
- Esophagogastric varices
- Mallory-Weiss tear from ↓ abdominal pressure (coughing, vomiting) ← esophageal wall rupture
- Neoplasms
- Liver disorders

Causes of lower GI bleeding include:

- Diverticulitis
- Infectious colitis, Crohn's disease
- Bowel disease or trauma, ischemic bowel
- Eroding aortic aneurysm
- Neoplasms and polyps
- Hemorrhoids or anorectal disorders

Pathophysiology

- Constriction of peripheral arteries → ↓ blood flow to skin and kidneys → renal failure; ↓ blood flow to GI tract → mesenteric insufficiency → bowel infarction and liver necrosis; ↓ blood flow to coronary arteries → myocardial infarction (MI); ↓ blood flow to brain → confusion, anxiety, restlessness, stupor, and coma.
- Acute massive GI bleeding → ↓ blood volume → ↓ venous return, ↓ cardiac output → ↑ HR, ↓ BP; ↑ HR → hypovolemic shock and multiple organ dysfunction.
- Metabolic acidosis and lactic acid accumulation ← anoxia and respiratory failure.

Clinical Presentation

- Hematemesis: Bright red or brown, coffee-ground emesis or NG tube drainage
- Melena: black, tarry stools
- Hematochezia: Maroon stools or bright red blood from rectum
- Hypotension: May be orthostatic, light-headedness, fainting. Orthostatic changes: ↓ BP >10 mm Hg with ↓ HR 20 bpm sitting or standing indicating volume depletion of 15% or more
- Tachycardia, ↑ pulse pressure, MAP <60 mm Hg, capillary refill sluggish

- Cardiac dysrhythmias
- Tachypnea, shortness of breath, chest pain
- Abdominal pain, rebound tenderness, or guarding
- Pallor, apprehension, confusion, lethargy, weakness
- ↓ urine output, ↑ urine concentration
- ↑ bowel sounds, diarrhea
- Cool, clammy skin and diaphoresis
- Stupor and coma if large blood loss
- Multiple organ dysfunction if severe blood loss (>30% blood volume) and hypovolemic shock

Diagnostic Tests

- CBC, platelets, and coagulation studies
- Basic metabolic profile (BMP), liver function tests, and BUN/creatinine ratio (if >36 → GI bleeding if no renal insufficiency)
- ECG to detect arrhythmias and/or cardiac enzymes if risk for MI
- ABGs or pulse oximetry
- UGI series
- Abdominal x-ray or CT of abdomen
- Barium enema
- GI bleeding scan. Calculate Rockall Score of Upper GI Bleeding at https://www.mdcalc.com/rockall-score-upper-gi-bleeding-complete or refer to GI Tab, Esophageal Varices
- Endoscopy including test for *Helicobacter pylori*
- Colonoscopy or sigmoidoscopy
- Mesenteric angiography

American College of Surgeons Classes of Acute Hemorrhage				
Factors	I	II	III	IV
Blood loss	<15% (<750 mL)	15%–30% (750–1,500 mL)	30%–40% (1,500–2,000 mL)	>40% (>2,000 mL)
Pulse	>100	>100	>120	>140
B.P.	Normal	Normal	↓	↓↓
Pulse pressure	N or ↓	↓	↓↓	↓↓

American College of Surgeons Classes of
Acute Hemorrhage—cont'd

Factors	I	II	III	IV
Capillary refill	<2 sec	2-3 sec	3-4 sec	>5 sec
Resp. rate	14-20	20-30	30-40	>40
Urine output mL/hr	30 or more	20-30	5-10	Negligible
Mental status	Slightly anxious	Mildly anxious	Anxious & confused	Confused Lethargic

From Committee on Trauma. Advanced Trauma Life Support Manual. Chicago: American College of Surgeons; 1997, pp. 103-112.

Management

■ Monitor vital signs and hemodynamics (central venous pressure [CVP], pulmonary artery pressure [PAP]). Arterial line recommended. Note ↑ BP, ↓ HR, ↑ CVP and cardiac output and other signs of shock. Treat shock symptoms. Type and crossmatch for 2-6 units of blood if transfusion needed, depending on rate of active bleeding.
■ Use ECG monitoring and assess for cardiac dysrhythmias.
■ Assess respiratory status and ABGs or pulse oximetry. Assess for signs of hypoxia. Administer O₂ via cannula, mask, or mechanical ventilation.
■ Consider NGT placement if indicated. Lavage as necessary with tap water or saline. Avoid iced lavage. Assess color and amount of drainage. Note bright red to coffee-ground drainage. Keep patient NPO if actively bleeding. Start clear liquids when bleeding stops. Keep head of bed elevated.
■ Place patient in left lateral decubitus position to ↑ risk of aspiration from acute bleeding.
■ Assess bowel sounds; assess abdomen for distention and palpate for pain.
■ Fluid resuscitation with two large-bore IV catheters or central access. Administer IV fluids (LR or NS), colloids, crystalloids, blood, and blood products. Administration of blood and blood products should be individualized to the patient's condition and hemodynamic status.
■ Note amount and color of feces. Hematest stool prn. Monitor CBC, PT, PTT, and blood chemistries.
■ Insert Foley catheter. Monitor intake and output. Assess fluid and electrolyte balance.

- Administer high-dose proton pump inhibitors to maintain gastric pH >6.0. Histamine antagonists are not recommended. Consider misoprostol (prostaglandin analog), anticholinergics, or mucosal protective agents.
- Administer IV or intra-arterial vasopressin (Pitressin) with caution. Consider octreotide (Sandostatin), terlipressin, ornipressin, or somatostatin, especially if varices suspected.
- If coagulopathy is present (↑ PTT), administer vitamin K 10 mg IV and fresh frozen plasma.
- Administer tranexamic acid (Cyklokapron) if excessive bleeding and decreased fibrinolysis.
- A specific protocol of medications is ordered if patient is *H. pylori* positive.
- Assess for hemorrhagic shock and estimate fluid and blood loss.
- Provide emotional support to patient and family. Relieve anxiety and pain.
- Prepare patient for possible endoscopic or surgical procedures:
    - Upper endoscopy; angiography may be helpful
    - Clips, thermocoagulation, or sclerosant injection should be used with epinephrine injection
    - Intra-arterial embolization
    - Vagotomy, pyloroplasty, or total or partial gastrectomy may be required

Complications

- Gastric perforation → sudden and severe generalized abdominal pain with rebound tenderness and board-like abdominal rigidity
- Reduced cardiac output, including hypovolemic shock. Kidney failure.
- Nausea, vomiting, and diarrhea; pulmonary aspiration
- Altered nutritional status with nutritional deficits and anemia; aspiration
- Infection; fever, ↑ WBC and ↑ HR; sepsis

Esophageal Varices

Esophageal varices are dilated, distended, tortuous veins in the esophagus. They may also occur in the proximal stomach. These varices most commonly result from portal hypertension (>10 mm Hg) secondary to hepatic cirrhosis caused by the consumption of large amounts of alcohol. Severe liver disease → blood coagulation abnormalities → bleeding.

Pathophysiology

Impaired liver structure and function → ↑ resistance to portal blood flow at portal vena and inferior vena cava and ↑ pressure in the liver → ↑ portal venous pressure (portal hypertension) → collateral circulation from the liver to the veins of the esophagus, spleen, intestines, and stomach → engorged and dilated blood vessels → esophagogastric varices → rupture → massive hemorrhage → death.

Clinical Presentation

- Vomiting of blood (hematemesis) or massive bleeding (hematochezia)
- Tachycardia; ↓ BP; cool, clammy skin; decreased urine output
- Bright red to black stools, indicating blood in feces
- Abdominal pain and weakness
- Other signs of UGI bleeding

Rockall Scoring System to Predict Mortality in Acute UGI Bleeding

Variable	Score of 0	Score of 1	Score of 2	Score of 3
Age (yr)	<60	60–79	≥80	
Shock	No shock HR <100 bpm SBP >100 mm Hg	HR >100 bpm SBP <100 mm Hg	HR >100 bpm SBP <100 mm Hg	
Comorbidity	No major comorbidity		Heart failure, ischemic heart disease, any major comorbidity	Renal failure, liver failure, metastatic cancer
Diagnosis	Mallory-Weiss tear, no pathology	All other diagnoses: e.g., esophagitis, gastritis, peptic ulcer disease, varices	Malignancy of UGI tract	
Endoscopic evidence of bleeding or recent hemorrhage	None or dark spot only		Blood in UGI tract, adherent clot, visible or spurting vessel	

Interpretation: Score <3 indicates good prognosis. Total score >8 indicates a high risk of mortality.

Diagnostic Tests

- Refer to Acute Gastrointestinal Bleeding for appropriate diagnostic tests.
- CBC, serum chemistries, and liver function tests
- Platelet count, PT/PTT, and fibrinogen
- Type and crossmatch for possible blood administration
- Endoscopy, ultrasound, CT, MRI, nuclear imaging
- Liver biopsy
- Angiography: Indirect arterial portography, percutaneous transhepatic portography (TIP), or hepatic phlebography

Management

- Administer antibiotics to prevent/control infection.
- Provide nutritional supplementation.
- Administer lactulose (Cephulac).
- Administer octreotide (Sandostatin) infusion to ↓ portal pressure. Usually given as a 50-mcg IV bolus followed with a drip at 25 mcg/hr. Consider administration of somatostatin, which has a shorter half-life and different hemodynamic effects than Sandostatin. Usually given as a 250 mcg IV bolus followed with a drip of 250 mcg/hr.
- Initiate arterial or central line infusion of vasopressin (Pitressin). Use with caution → myocardial or mesenteric ischemia and infarction because of vasoconstriction.
- Insert esophagogastric balloon tamponade.
- Prepare patient for endoscopic variceal ligation or endoscopic sclerotherapy.
- Prepare patient for transjugular intrahepatic portosystemic shunt (TIPS) or endoscopic injection. Percutaneous TIPS is an interventional procedure to decrease portal hypertension and reduce complications of high hepatic pressures. A catheter is placed in a hepatic vein, and a stent is placed in the liver parenchyma. After the procedure: Observe for bleeding from hepatic or portal vein puncture, puncture of the biliary tree, bile duct trauma, and stent migration or thrombosis.
- Refer to assessment and management discussions in Acute Gastrointestinal Bleeding.

Esophagogastric Balloon Tamponade

- Esophagogastric balloon tamponade is used to control esophageal variceal bleeding through use of the Sengstaken-Blakemore tube or Minnesota tube. A Linton-Nachlas tube is used for isolated gastric hemorrhage, such as with gastric varices. The balloons apply direct pressure to the varices → ↓ blood flow and stop variceal bleeding.

- The Sengstaken-Blakemore tube has three lumens: gastric aspiration, esophageal balloon inflation, and gastric balloon inflation. The Minnesota tube has a fourth lumen for esophageal aspiration. The inflation of the balloons is as follows or per policy:
  - The esophageal balloon is inflated to 25–35/40 mm Hg pressure for a maximum of 24 hr. Note pressure on manometer.
  - The gastric balloon is inflated in 100-mL increments to 25–500 mL of air or as specified by manufacturer. Note pressure on manometer.
  - Never inflate the esophageal balloon before the gastric balloon.
  - 1–3 lb of pressure is used for tension or traction on the balloons by using a pulley system with a 500-mL bag of IV fluid, a football helmet, or a foam rubber cuff.
  - One port is connected to intermittent suction.

Nursing Management of Esophageal Balloon Tamponade

- Confirm placement by chest x-ray.
- Assess airway patency and signs of respiratory distress. Sudden rupture of balloon → airway obstruction and pulmonary aspiration of gastric contents and asphyxiation.
- Scissors should be placed at the bedside for cutting the balloons if airway is obstructed.
- Position patient in high-Fowler's position or on left side.
- Provide frequent oral and nares care and oral suction.
- Monitor lumen pressures, cardiac rhythm, VS, and respiratory status.
- Consider sedation or restraints.
- An optional NG tube may be inserted along the course of the Sengstaken-Blakemore tube with the tip of the NG tube 3–4 cm proximal to the esophageal balloon.
- Monitor gastric and esophageal output. Maintain suction on ports. The balloons may be deflated for about 30 min every 8–12 hr or per policy to decompress the esophagus and stomach. Assess for bleeding.
  - The esophageal balloon must be deflated before the gastric balloon to prevent upward migration of the esophageal balloon → airway occlusion.
- To discontinue tamponade therapy, gradually decrease esophageal balloon pressure. Observe for bleeding. If no further bleeding, then deflate the gastric balloon. If no further bleeding within the following 4 hr, the tube may be removed. Continue to monitor for bleeding.

Complications

- Esophageal erosion and rupture → bleeding and shock
- Pulmonary aspiration
- Balloon migration resulting in asphyxiation

- Nasal necrosis and mucosal ulceration
- Hiccups

Institution-specific care:

- _____
- _____
- _____
- _____
- _____

Liver Failure

Liver or hepatic failure occurs when 60% of hepatocytes are lost. It may be chronic or acute and can lead to hepatic encephalopathy or hepatic coma. Causes of liver failure include:

- Cirrhosis of the liver
- Hepatitis A, hepatitis B, hepatitis C, Epstein-Barr virus, and other viral infections
- IV drug use, cocaine use, and acetaminophen toxicity
- Repeated environmental and hepatotoxin exposure
- Malignancy
- Hypoperfusion of the liver
- Metabolic disorders: Reye's syndrome, Wilson's disease
- Autoimmune disorders
- Malnutrition, diabetes mellitus, chronic cholestatic disease, and hypertriglyceridemia
- Postoperatively: jejunoileal bypass, partial hepatectomy, liver transplant failure

Pathophysiology

- Severe liver impairment such as necrosis or ↓ blood supply to liver → toxic substances accumulating in the blood.
- Impaired bilirubin conjugation, ↓ clotting factors, ↓ glucose synthesis, ↓ lactate clearance → jaundice, coagulopathies, hypoglycemia, and metabolic acidosis.
- Decreased macrophages in liver → ↑ risk of infection and spleen enlargement.
- Hypoalbuminemia, fluid and electrolyte imbalances, acute portal hypertension → development of ascites.

GI

- Ineffective fat metabolism ← ↑ bile salt production.
- Cirrhosis: Fibrotic tissue replaces healthy liver tissue.
- Fatty liver disease: Fatty cells replace healthy liver tissue.
- Hepatic failure may progress to hepatic encephalopathy.

Clinical Presentation

- Jaundice and pruritus, ascites, edema, JVD
- Right upper quadrant tenderness or abdominal pain
- Malnutrition, nausea, vomiting, hematemesis, melena, and anorexia
- Weakness, fatigue, and confusion. Increased intracranial pressure
- Hyperventilation, respiratory alkalosis, dyspnea, pleural effusion, crackles, and hypoxemia
- Hypokalemia and hyponatremia or hypernatremia
- Palmar erythema, spider nevi, spider angiomas, and bruising; patient prone to bleeding
- Asterixis: Liver flap (patient extends arms ← wrist dorsiflexes downward involuntarily)
- Metabolic acidosis, hypoglycemia, hypokalemia, and hyponatremia
- Gallstones, urine malnutrition, light or clay-colored stools, and dark urine
- Diarrhea and steatorrhea (fatty, greasy, foul-smelling stools)
- Hepatic encephalopathy; Drowsiness, confusion, delirium or coma, inappropriate behavior, fetor hepaticus (sweet, slightly fecal breath odor), and day-night reversal

Diagnostic Tests

- CT scan or ultrasound
- Serum chemistries, bilirubin, total protein, and albumin
- AST, APT, ALT, and cholesterol
- Ammonia and lactate levels
- CBC and platelets
- ABGs or pulse oximetry
- ECG to detect arrhythmias
- PT, PTT, INR, plasmin, plasminogen, fibrin, and fibrin-split products
- Urinalysis, urine bilirubin, and urine urobilinogen
- EEG to assess brain function if indicated
- Drug screening as appropriate
- Liver biopsy may be needed if not contraindicated

Management

- Administer lactulose (Cephulac) orally or rectally to ↓ ammonia levels.
- Administer neomycin orally or rectally if not contraindicated.
- Administer diuretics such as furosemide (Lasix) if ascites present. Monitor intake and output. Measure abdominal girth.
- A pulmonary artery catheter may be needed to monitor hemodynamics.
- Prepare patient for paracentesis if necessary.
- Monitor for cardiac dysrhythmias.
- Provide stress ulcer prophylaxis. Elevate head of bed 20°–30°. Assess for signs of GI bleeding. Gastric suction as necessary.
- Administer vitamin K and platelets. Use bleeding precautions. Avoid frequent venipunctures.
- Administer thiamine, riboflavin, pyridoxine, folic acid.
- Treat fever and control BP. Consider dopamine or norepinephrine if hypotension.
- Correct fluid and electrolyte imbalances. Prevent and correct hypokalemia, which increases renal ammonia production → ammonia across the blood-brain barrier. Avoid lactated Ringer's solution.
- Prevent infection. Administer prophylactic antibiotics. Consider rifaximin (Xifaxan) or metronidazole (Flagyl).
- Assess neurological status including mental status, level of consciousness, Glasgow Coma Scale score, and response to verbal and noxious stimuli.
- Assess for signs of ICP. Administer mannitol if indicated.
- Consider sorbitol-induced catharsis to prevent osmotic diarrhea.
- Assess respiratory status, and monitor ABGs or pulse oximetry. Correct hypercapnia and hypoxemia via O_2 administration or mechanical ventilation.
- Provide CRRT if renal failure present.
- Avoid benzodiazepines and other sedatives that may mask symptoms. Consider oxazepam (Serax), diazepam (Valium), or lorazepam (Ativan) if sedation is required.
- Administer flumazenil (Romazicon), a benzodiazepine antagonist, if necessary.
- Use physical restraints as necessary. Provide reality orientation. Institute measures for patient safety.
- Administer medications with caution. Adjust dosage per liver function tests.
- Provide a low-protein, low-sodium diet. Restrict fluids as necessary. Consider enteral feeding or TPN if oral intake insufficient. Assess for hypoglycemia. Monitor serum albumin, electrolytes, and liver function tests. IV glucose may minimize protein breakdown. Monitor glucose levels.

- Prevent intravascular volume depletion through IV fluids, colloids, and crystalloids. Avoid lactated Ringer's solution.
- Avoid hazards of immobility. Provide meticulous skin care.
- Monitor ammonia levels (80–110 mcg/dL or 47–65 mcmol/L [SI units] is normal).
- Provide comfort measures and emotional support.
- Prepare patient for liver transplantation if necessary. Calculate a MELD score (Model for End-Stage Liver Disease) for transplant patient selection. Refer to https://optn.transplant.hrsa.gov/resources/allocation-calculators/meld-calculator/ or https://www.mdcalc.com/meld-score-model-end-stage-liver-disease-12-older
- Prepare patient for TIPS to ↑ portal hypertension, prevent rebleeding from varices, and ↑ formation of ascites or shunt surgery if indicated. Refer to management under Esophageal Varices.

Complications

- Cerebral edema and increased ICP, and low cerebral perfusion pressure
- Cardiac dysrhythmias and coagulopathy
- Respiratory depression, acute respiratory failure, and respiratory arrest
- Sepsis and circulatory failure
- Acute renal failure
- Hypoxemia, metabolic acidosis, and electrolyte imbalances
- Hypoglycemia
- GI bleeding
- Hepatic failure may progress to **hepatic encephalopathy** ← **death**.
- Hepatic encephalopathy is divided into the following types:
  - **Type A:** Hepatic encephalopathy associated with acute liver failure
  - **Type B:** Hepatic encephalopathy caused by portosystemic shunting without associated intrinsic liver disease
  - **Type C:** Hepatic encephalopathy associated with cirrhosis
- The severity of hepatic encephalopathy is evaluated according to the following grades:
  - Grade 1: Euphoria or anxiety, shortened attention span
  - Grade 2: Lethargy, apathy, subtle personality change, inappropriate behavior, minimal disorientation to time or place
  - Grade 3: Somnolence to semistupor, response to verbal stimuli, confusion
  - Grade 4: Coma, lack of response to stimuli

Acute Pancreatitis

Pancreatitis is an inflammation of the pancreas that can be categorized as edematous interstitial pancreatitis or acute necrotizing pancreatitis; 10%–20% of cases of pancreatitis are idiopathic and have no etiologic factor. Causes of pancreatitis include:

- Alcohol abuse
- Gallstones, biliary tract disease, hypercholesteremia, hypertriglyceridemia
- Pancreatic cysts, abscess, necrosis, or tumors
- Infection (e.g., mumps, ischemia)
- Blunt abdominal trauma and surgical trauma
- Hyperparathyroidism, hypercalcemia, and hyperthyroidism
- Systemic lupus erythematosus and vasculitis
- Medications such as glucocorticoids, sulfonamides, tetracyclines, NSAIDs, furosemide, procainamide, hydrochlorothiazide, ACE inhibitors, valproic acid, and estrogen

Pathophysiology

- Trypsinogen is converted to trypsin (pancreatic enzymes) → destruction of ductal tissue and pancreatic cells → autodigestion and fibrosis of the pancreas.
- An increase in capillary permeability → leakage of fluid into the interstitium → edema, hypovolemia, hemorrhage, pancreatic, and adipose tissue necrosis → third spacing of fluids → systemic inflammatory response syndrome (SIRS).
- Obstruction of the pancreatic duct → reflux of bile into the pancreas → enzyme reaction.
- Drugs and toxins → autodigestion and inflammation.

Clinical Presentation

- Severe knife-like midepigastric or midabdominal pain that may radiate to the back; onset of pain frequently 24–48 hr after a heavy meal or alcohol ingestion; pain possibly also diffuse and difficult to localize
- Nausea and vomiting, anorexia
- Fever, diaphoresis, and weakness
- Tachypnea, ↓ BP, ↑ HR, and other symptoms of hypovolemic shock or respiratory distress
- Hypoactive or absent bowel sounds, and abdominal tenderness and distention
- Ascites and jaundice if illness severe

- Steatorrhea: Fatty, foul-smelling stools
- Pancreatic hemorrhage → Grey Turner's sign (gray-blue discoloration of the flank) or Cullen's sign (discoloration of the umbilical region)
- Palpable abdominal mass if pseudocyst or abscess present
- Hypocalcemia causing twitching and seizures; hyperlipidemia
- Restlessness, mental confusion, agitation

Ranson's Criteria for Predicting Mortality in Pancreatitis

Assessment completed on admission and again in 48 hr.

On Admission		48 Hours After Admission	
Age >55 y.o.	1 point	Hct decrease >10%	1 point
WBC >16,000 cells/mm^2	1 point	BUN >5 mg/dL after IV hydration	1 point
Serum glucose >200 mg/dL	1 point	Serum calcium <8 mg/dL	1 point
Serum LDH >350 IUnits/L	1 point	Arterial PO$_2$ <60 mm Hg	1 point
Serum AST (SGOT) >250 IUnits/mL	1 point	Base deficit >4 mEq/L	1 point
		Fluid sequestration/ needs >6 L	1 point

- Score of <3   predicted mortality 1%
- Score of 3–4   predicted mortality 15%
- Score of 5–6   predicted mortality 40%
- Score of >6   predicted mortality 100%

Diagnostic Tests

- Serum amylase (30–220 Units/L [SI units] normal) and/or lipase (0–160 Units/L [SI units] normal) more than three times the upper limit of normal
- Serum lactate
- Abdominal flat plate radiograph or ultrasound of abdomen, CT, MRI, and endoscopic cholangiopancreatography
- Chest x-ray to detect pleural effusions
- Serum chemistries, including ↑ calcium, ↑ magnesium, ↓ bilirubin, ↓ glucose, ↑ potassium, ↓ albumin, ↓ triglycerides, and ↓ liver enzymes, ↑ lipase

- Urinalysis and ↑ urinary amylase (6.5–48.1 Units/hr [SI units] normal)
- CBC (↑ WBC, hematocrit and hemoglobin may be ↑ or ↓), PT/PTT, ↑ C-reactive protein
- ABGs to assess for hypoxemia and metabolic acidosis
- ECG – ST-segment depression and T-wave inversion

Management

- Administer analgesics; position patient in knee-chest position.
- Consider prophylactic antibiotics. For necrotizing pancreatitis, administer imipenem-cilastatin (Primaxin) for its high concentration of the drug in the pancreas.
- Assess fluid and electrolyte balance. Note hypokalemia, hypomagnesemia, or hypocalcemia. Administer IV fluids, crystalloids, and colloids. Monitor intake and output.
- Assess nutritional status. Keep patient NPO initially. Consider TPN or gastric or jejunal enteral feedings. Stress ulcer prophylaxis.
- Insert NG tube if vomiting, obstruction, or gastric distention is present. Provide frequent oral care.
- Assess for metabolic acidosis.
- Assess neurological status for confusion and lethargy.
- Assess respiratory status and monitor ABGs or venous oxygen saturation. Administer O_2 as needed. Prevent ARDS from loss of surfactant.
- Administer insulin if elevated blood glucose levels exist.
- Assess abdomen for distention, rigidity, ascites, and increasing pain or rebound tenderness; auscultate bowel sounds and measure abdominal girth.
- Administer anticholinergics, pantoprazole (Protonix) or famotidine (Pepcid) as indicated.
- Treat fever and monitor WBC count.
- Assess vital signs. Monitor for cardiac arrhythmias.
- Prepare patient for surgical débridement or pancreatic resection for necrotizing pancreatitis or drainage of pancreatic pseudocyst or abscess or Whipple's procedure.

Complications

- Pancreatic abscess, necrosis or pseudocyst formation, and bowel infarction
- Acute lung injury (ALI), ARDS, pleural effusion, atelectasis, pneumonia, pneumonitis, hypoxemia, and respiratory failure
- Hypotension, pericardial effusion, myocardial depression, heart failure, cardiac dysrhythmias, and DIC
- Acute renal failure, acute tubular necrosis, and azotemia
- Hepatic dysfunction, obstructive jaundice, and paralytic ileus

- Long-term insulin dependence and frequent exacerbations
- Stress ulcers and esophageal varices → GI hemorrhage
- SIRS
- Severe hemorrhage and shock
- Multiorgan failure, sepsis, and death

Peritonitis

Peritonitis is inflammation of the peritoneum, the serous membrane lining the abdominal cavity and covering the viscera. It may be localized or generalized. Peritonitis is an example of acute abdomen.

Pathophysiology

Inflammation, bacterial infection, ischemia, tumor, and trauma → leakage of contents from the abdominal organs into the abdominal cavity → proliferation of bacteria → tissue edema → fluid in peritoneal cavity.

Clinical Presentation

- Abdominal pain that increases with movement such as coughing and flexing the hips; rebound tenderness, guarding, and abdominal rigidity (washboard abdomen); Blumberg's sign: Pressing a hand on the abdomen elicits pain, but pain increases when releasing the hand as the peritoneum moves back into place
- Air and fluid in the bowel
- Abdominal distention, hyperactive → hypoactive bowel sounds → paralytic ileus
- Nausea and vomiting, anorexia
- Fever, chills and ↓ HR
- Worsening or new onset of renal failure
- Cloudy effluent if patient undergoing peritoneal dialysis

Diagnostic Tests

- CBC: Assess for leukocytosis, and ↑ hemoglobin and hematocrit
- Serum chemistries
- Abdominal x-ray, CT abdomen, MRI
- Peritoneal lavage or peritoneal aspiration and C&S studies of peritoneal fluid or peritoneal effluent

Complications

- Fluid and electrolyte imbalance, ↓ CVP, hypovolemia → shock → acute renal failure
- Intestinal obstruction from bowel adhesions
- Peritoneal abscess
- Sepsis

Management

- Administer antibiotics. Obtain blood cultures to assess for sepsis.
- Obtain peritoneal effluent cultures.
- Provide fluid and electrolyte replacement. Administer colloids. Monitor intake and output.
- Use gastric or intestinal tubes to suction as indicated.
- Administer analgesics and antiemetics. Place patient on side with knees flexed.
- Monitor vital signs. Assess for ↓ BP and ↑ HR. Provide cardiac monitoring.
- Assess respiratory status. Administer O_2 or ventilator assistance as indicated by ABGs or pulse oximetry.
- Assess abdomen for pain and distention. Auscultate bowel sounds.
- Prepare patient for surgery as indicated to remove infected material and correct the cause.
- Complications include wound evisceration and abscess formation.

Crohn's Disease

Crohn's disease is an inflammatory bowel disease that may occur anywhere along the GI tract. The terminal ileum and proximal large intestine are usually involved.

Pathophysiology

Chronic inflammation → edema and thickening of intestinal mucosa → ulcers forming in the intestines → fistulas, fissures, and abscesses → thickening of bowel wall → narrowing of intestinal lumen → scar tissue and granulomas → weepy edematous intestines.

Clinical Presentation

- Lower right quadrant crampy abdominal pain that usually occurs after meals
- Abdominal tenderness and spasm
- Chronic diarrhea and steatorrhea (excessive fat in stool)
- Weight loss, anorexia, malnutrition, anemia, and nutritional deficiencies

Diagnostic Tests

- Sigmoidoscopy, colonoscopy, intestinal biopsies, and testing for *Clostridium difficile*
- Stool analysis for occult blood and steatorrhea and stool C&S
- UGI series or endoscopy and barium enema/series
- Abdominal x-rays and CT, MRI, or ultrasound of the abdomen
- CBC, ESR, and C-reactive protein
- Serum chemistries, including albumin, protein, and calcium, and liver function tests

Management

- Administer 5-aminosalicylic acid derivatives:
  - Mesalamine or mesalazine (5-ASA, Asacol, Pentasa)
  - Balsalazide (Colazal)
- Administer corticosteroids:
  - Prednisone or hydrocortisone
  - Prednisolone or methylprednisolone
  - Budesonide
- Consider administration of antibiotics such as metronifazole (Flagyl) or ciprofloacin (Cipro).
- Consider: natalizumab (Tysabri), infliximab (Remicade), adallmumab (humira), certollzumab pegol (cimzia), ustekinumab (stelara) azathioprine (Imuran), mercaptopurine (6-MP), methotrexate, or tacrollmus.
- Administer analgesics for pain such as anticholinergics.
- Assess vital signs for ↑ HR and fever, and assess for pallor.
- Assess bowel sounds, and examine abdomen for distention and tenderness.
- Assess number and frequency of stools, and test stool for occult blood and parasites. Administer antidiarrheals such as loperamide (Imodium) or diphenoxylate-atropine (Lomotil) or bile acid sequestrants such as cholestyramine or colestipol. Consider bulk hydrophilic agents.

- Administer IV fluids to correct fluid and electrolyte imbalance.
- Maintain NPO with TPN, or provide diet high in protein and calories with vitamins and iron.
- Prepare patient for surgery as needed (partial or complete colectomy with ileostomy of anastomosis).

Complications

- Abscesses, fistulas and sinus tracts, strictures, adhesions
- Small bowel obstruction or bowel perforation
- Right-sided hydronephrosis
- Cholelithiasis
- Toxic megacolon

Ulcerative Colitis

Ulcerative colitis is an inflammatory autoimmune disease of the bowel. It is characterized by ulcers or open sores in the colon that affect the mucosal layer. The patient experiences remissions and exacerbations and has an increased risk of colorectal cancer.

Pathophysiology

Multiple ulcerations of the colon → bleeding → mucosa becomes edematous and inflamed → abscesses → narrowing, shortening and thickening of the bowel.

Clinical Presentation

- Diarrhea mixed with blood and mucus (as many as 10–20 liquid stools/day) and an urgent need to defecate
- Crampy abdominal pain in the left lower quadrant and rebound tenderness in the right lower quadrant
- Intermittent tenesmus: Constant feeling of the need to defecate with little or no fecal output
- Rectal bleeding
- Pallor, anemia, and fatigue
- Anorexia, weight loss, vomiting, and dehydration
- Fever and tachycardia

Diagnostic Tests

- Sigmoidoscopy, colonoscopy, intestinal biopsies, and testing for C. difficile
- Stool analysis for occult blood and steatorrhea and stool C&S
- UGI series or endoscopy and barium enema
- Abdominal x-rays and CT, MRI, or ultrasound of the abdomen
- CBC, ESR, and C-reactive protein
- Serum chemistries, including albumin, protein, and calcium, and liver function tests

Management

- Assess vital signs for ↑ HR, ↓ BP, ↑ RR, and fever, and assess for pallor.
- Assess skin in the perianal area for redness and skin breakdown.
- Assess bowel sounds, and examine abdomen for distention and tenderness.
- Assess number and frequency of stools, and test stool for occult blood and parasites.
- Administer IV fluids to correct fluid and electrolyte imbalance.
- Maintain NPO with TPN, or provide diet high in protein and calories with vitamins and iron.
- Administer bulk hydrophilic agents and antidiarrheals.
- Administer antibiotics, 5-aminosalicylate derivates, corticosteroids and other anti-inflammatory medications. Refer to Crohn's disease, GI Tab.
- Prepare patient for surgery as needed (total colectomy with ileostomy, continent ileostomy, or bowel resection).

Complications

- Toxic megacolon → colonic distention → fever, abdominal pain and distention, vomiting, and fatigue (does not respond to medical management within 24–72 hr); total colectomy possibly indicated
- Intestinal perforation and bleeding; intra-abdominal abscesses, fistulas, strictures
- Pyelonephritis and nephrolithiasis
- Malignant neoplasms

Small Bowel Obstruction (SBO)

SBO is a mechanical or functional obstruction of the small intestines. The normal transit of the products of digestion through the intestines is blocked.

Causes

- Adhesions, hernias, volvulus, intussusception, strictures, abscess, paralytic ileus
- Crohn's disease
- Benign or malignant tumors
- Foreign bodies

Pathophysiology

- Intestinal contents, gas, and fluid accumulate above the obstruction → abdominal distention and fluid retention → ↓ venous and arteriolar capillary pressure → edema, congestion of the intestine → rupture or perforation of the intestinal wall → peritonitis. ↓ blood supply to obstruction → ischemia → necrosis and gangrene of the intestine. Obstruction may be partial or complete and may also lead to intestinal strangulation.
- Reflex vomiting also occurs → ↓ H^+ and K^+ → metabolic acidosis, and ↓ H_2O and ↓ Na^+ → dehydration → hypovolemic shock.
- Obstruction may resolve spontaneously.

Clinical Presentation

- Crampy, colicky, wave-like central or midabdominal pain
- No bowel movement and absence of flatus → abdominal distention → bowel ischemia or perforation
- Nausea and vomiting → dehydration (drowsiness, malaise, parched tongue and mucous membranes, intense thirst) and electrolyte imbalances → hypovolemic shock
- Possible aspiration of vomitus (vomitus may be fecal in nature)

Diagnostic Tests

- Abdominal x-ray, CT scan, and ultrasound of the abdomen
- Contrast enema or small bowel series
- Colonoscopy and laparoscopy
- CBC and serum chemistries

Management

- Insert NG tube and connect to low intermittent suction; assess color and amount of drainage.

- Administer IV fluids, and assess fluid and electrolyte balance.
- Monitor nutritional status. Monitor intake and output.
- Assess abdomen for bowel sounds, pain, and distention.
- Administer analgesics for pain.
- Prepare patient for surgery as indicated to relieve the obstruction. Acute complete SBO is a surgical emergency.

Bowel Infarction or Acute Mesenteric Ischemia

Pathophysiology

Decreased blood supply to bowel and mesenteric circulation → ischemia → gangrene of bowel wall → bowel infarction.

Clinical Presentation

- Severe acute abdominal pain
- Bloody stools with diarrhea
- Fever
- Nausea and vomiting, abdominal distention with guarding and tenderness

Diagnostic Tests

- CBC with elevated WBC
- Barium enema, colonoscopy
- Abdominal x-ray, CT of abdomen, ultrasound of abdomen

Management

- Surgical treatment may include colostomy or ileostomy.
- Complications include peritonitis, sepsis, and acute renal failure.
- DVT prophylaxis important.

Intra-Abdominal Hypertension (IAH) or Abdominal Compartment Syndrome (ACS)

IAH is characterized by an increase in abdominal pressure caused primarily by abdominal trauma, major burns, ruptured aortic aneurysm, mechanical intestinal obstruction, abdominal operations with tight closures, or intraperitoneal diseases such as severe pancreatitis, intra-abdominal infection, ascites, abdominal tumors, or sepsis. It may lead to the development of abdominal compartment syndrome, shock, multiple organ failure, and death.

Pathophysiology

Compression of intestinal tract → thrombosis and bowel wall edema → fluid accumulation and ↑ intra-abdominal pressure (IAP) → ↓ arterial blood flow to abdominal organs → ischemia and anaerobic metabolism.

Normal IAP = 0–5 mm Hg. Mean IAP in critically ill adults = 5–7 mm Hg.
IAH is sustained/repeated ↑ of IAP >12 mm Hg.
Abdominal perfusion pressure (APP) = MAP – IAP. Maintain at >60 mm Hg.
An increase IAP to 20 mm Hg → ↓ in mesenteric perfusion by 40%. IAP 40 mm Hg → ↓ mesenteric perfusion by 70%.

Clinical Presentation

- Wheezes, crackles, tachypnea, respiratory distress
- Increase in abdominal girth
- Syncope
- Decreased urine output
- Nausea, vomiting, melena
- Signs and symptoms of multiple organ failure

Diagnostic Tests

- Primarily by abdominal CT or abdominal ultrasound
- Abdominal x-rays of little value

Management

- IAP monitoring using the trans-bladder technique. (Refer to World Society of the Abdominal Compartment Syndrome at http://www.wsacs.org)
- Fluid resuscitation
- Paracentesis
- Diuretics: furosemide (Lasix), spironolactone (Aldactone), amiloride (Midamor)
- Laparoscopic decompression
- Surgery possibly indicated to correct the underlying problem

Complications

- Renal failure
- Respiratory failure
- Bowel ischemia
- Shock
- Multisystem organ failure and death

Gastrointestinal Surgery With Anastomosis

Anastomosis of the GI system is a surgical procedure connecting two parts of the GI system. These include esophagectomy, Whipple's procedure, gastrojejunostomy, intestinal anastomosis including anastomosis involved in bariatric surgical procedures.

Complications

- Gastritis, esophagitis, dumping syndrome, peritonitis, and GI bleeding
- Anastomotic leak: Tachycardia, tachypnea, fever, abdominal pain, anxiety and restlessness, subcutaneous emphysema (crepitus), and sepsis
- Hepatorenal failure

Management

- Provide standard postoperative care, including administration of analgesics and provision of pulmonary care.
- Assess for GI bleeding.
- Provide DVT prophylaxis. Encourage early ambulation. Dietary restrictions per procedure.

Hematological and Oncological Disorders

Disseminated Intravascular Coagulation (DIC)

DIC is a disorder characterized by massive systemic intravascular activation of the coagulation cascade caused by a variety of clinical conditions, including sepsis (gram-positive and gram-negative infections), severe trauma or burns, solid or hematological cancers, organ destruction (i.e., pancreatitis), severe transfusion reactions, and vascular abnormalities. It can also be caused by some obstetrical conditions, such as placental abruption, amniotic fluid embolism, placenta previa, and retained dead fetus syndrome.

Pathophysiology

- Activation of thrombus → fibrinogen fibrin formation and deposition of fibrin in the microvasculature → an ↑ in platelet aggregation or adhesions → formation of fibrin clots to form → diffuse obstruction of the smaller vessels → progressive organ dysfunction (i.e., renal insufficiency, ARDS, hypotension, circulatory failure, skin necrosis).
- Concurrent with these events, platelets, prothrombin, and fibrinogen are depleted → a deficiency of these factors compromising coagulation and predisposing to bleeding.
- The excessive clotting at the microvasculature level activates the fibrinolytic system → production of fibrin degradation products (FDPs) (i.e., fibrin split products) → an anticoagulation effect of FDP with fibrinogen and thrombin → interference with the formation of fibrin clot and decreased platelet function → bleeding → hemorrhagic bleeding.

Clinical Presentation

- Bleeding (purpura, petechiae, ecchymosis). Bleeding from at least three unrelated sites is highly suggestive of DIC
- GI bleeding (hematemesis, melena, tarry stools)
- GU/GYN bleeding (hematuria, menorrhagia in women) and oliguria
- Wound bleeding
- Bleeding and oozing from puncture sites and around invasive catheters and lines
- Hematoma formation
- Dyspnea, hemoptysis, cough, pulmonary hemorrhage or hypoxia
- Signs of renal dysfunction or failure
- Large foci of skin necrosis (resulting from tissue injury and necrosis associated with compromised circulation)
- Acrocyanosis (cyanosis of hands and feet)
- Acute multiorgan dysfunction (characterized by hypotension, tachycardia, oliguria, dyspnea, confusion, convulsions, coma, abdominal pain, diarrhea, and other GI symptoms)

HEMA/
ONCO

- Palpitations
- Angina
- Malaise, fatigue, and weakness
- Acidosis
- Headache
- Nausea and vomiting
- Severe pain in abdomen, back, muscles, joints, and bones
- Sudden vision changes
- Vertigo
- Confusion and anxiety or irritability
- Convulsions
- Coma

Diagnostic Tests

- CBC (trend platelet counts)
- BUN and creatinine, bilirubin
- ABGs
- PT, PTT, INR
- Fibrinogen level
- Fibrin degradation/split products
- D-dimer assay
- Thrombin time
- Antithrombin III (AT III)
- Blood smear (schistocytes present)
- Factor V and factor VII
- Protein C and protein S level
- The International Society on Thrombosis and Haemostasis DIC Scoring System can be found at https://reference.medscape.com/calculator/dic-score

Management

- Treat underlying cause, if it can be treated.
- Be aware of early signs of impaired tissue perfusion in patients at high risk for DIC (subtle mental status change, hypotension [especially orthostatic], dyspnea, tachypnea, syncope, decreased urine output. Consider
- Monitor cardiac, respiratory, and neurological status.
- Assess for abnormal bleeding, and apply pressure to injection sites for at least 15 min.
- Monitor O₂ saturation and ABGs. Administer O₂ or mechanical ventilation as indicated. Sedation, antipyretics, and pain control to decrease O₂ demand.
- Administer IV fluids as needed.
- Monitor intake and output and signs of fluid overload.
- Consider heparin infusion or DVT prophylaxis with enoxaparin.
- Institute bleeding precautions.
- Replace deficient clotting factors.

202

- Administer vitamin K and folate.
- Consider platelet infusions.
- Administer fresh frozen plasma (FFP) infusion and packed RBCs.
- Consider cryoprecipitate (factor VIII) infusion.
- Provide blood transfusion and monitor for reactions.
- Provide support to patient and family.
- Assess for thrombotic and hemorrhagic conditions. Monitor for complications such as pulmonary embolism (PE), airway obstruction, acute tubular necrosis, increased ICP, or multiple organ failure and shock.

Heparin-Induced Thrombocytopenia (HIT)

HIT is a transient disorder in which thrombocytopenia (>50% ↓ in platelet count) appears 7–10 days after exposure to heparin. There is a strong association with venous and arterial blood clot formation. HIT is a thrombotic, not a bleeding, process.

Pathophysiology

After heparin is administered, an immune complex can form between heparin and specific blood factor (platelet factor 4 [PF4]) that is released by platelets → body viewing this "heparin-PF4" as a foreign body → formation of antibodies against the heparin PF4 complex → antibodies binding to the complex → platelet destruction → disruption of platelets → formation of new blood clot → deep vein thrombosis (DVT) or arterial occlusion, PE, myocardial infarction (MI), or cerebrovascular accident (CVA).

Clinical Presentation

- Signs and symptoms of DVT (pain or tenderness, sudden swelling, discoloration of visible leg veins) or manifestation of venous thrombus
- Signs and symptoms of PE (shortness of breath, change in HR, sharp chest pain, dizziness, anxiety, excessive sweating)
- Acute limb ischemia (from peripheral arterial occlusion)
- Venous limb gangrene (distal ischemic necrosis following DVT)
- Cerebral sinus thrombosis
- Manifestation of arterial thrombosis (less common)
- Stroke
- MI
- Organ infarction (kidney, mesentery)
- Fall in platelet count of >50% 5–10 days after initiation of heparin therapy
- Severe indicators:
  - Skin changes (bruising or blackening around injection site as well as on fingers, toes, and nipples), ↑ gangrene

HEMA/ONCO

Diagnostic Tests
- The serotonin release assay (SRA) is considered a diagnostic gold standard given its high sensitivity and specificity. However, because of its higher cost, the ELISA assay/PF4 is usually recommended first
- Platelet count, platelet aggregation, and platelet antibody screen
- Fibrinogen, fibrin degradation products, fibrin split products, and fibrin breakdown products
- Heparin-induced platelet aggregation assay
- Platelet activation assay (C-SRA; heparin-induced platelet activation assay)

Management
- Discontinue all heparin products. Avoid invasive procedures. If needed, apply pressure to site at least 5 min.
- Administer IV direct thrombin inhibitor for anticoagulation: argatroban.
- Monitor platelet count.
- Limit platelet infusions. Platelet transfusions may be needed if platelet count is low or spontaneous bleeding occurs.
- Once platelet count has increased to at least 150,000/mcL AND the patient has been stably anticoagulated with a thrombin-specific inhibitor, initiate Coumadin therapy. Dose should be tailored to maintain INR 2–3
- Provide a complete skin and neurovascular assessment.
- Assess for bleeding from lungs, GI and GU tracts, and brain.
- Review patient's medication list to avoid aspirin-containing products, NSAIDs, and antiplatelet agents.
- Provide support to patient and family.
- If a diagnosis of HIT has been made, heparin "allergy" should be included in patient's record, and a sign should be posted at bedside.
- For Guidelines on the Evaluation and Management of Adults with Suspected Heparin-Induced Thrombocytopenia (HIT): www.hematology.org/Clinicians/Guidelines-Quality/Quick-Ref/529.aspx
- A vena cava filter may be necessary to prevent pulmonary emboli.

Neutropenia

Neutropenia is an abnormally low absolute neutrophil count.

Pathophysiology
- Neutropenia is caused by neutrophil production and/or problems with neutrophil distribution as a result of infection, treatment, or drugs:
  - *Decreased production of neutrophils* caused by aplastic anemia, medications or toxins, metastatic cancer, lymphoma or leukemia, myelodysplastic syndrome, chemotherapy, or radiation

- *Increased destruction of neutrophils* (medication induced), resulting from immunological disease (e.g., systemic lupus erythematosus), viral disease (e.g., infectious hepatitis, mononucleosis), or bacterial infection
- Interruption of neutrophil production or neutrophil distribution → decrease in neutrophil count

Clinical Presentation

When a patient is neutropenic, the following usual signs of infection may not be present because of the lack of sufficient number of neutrophils needed to produce common infectious signs:

- Local warmth
- Local swelling
- Shaking chills

Common presenting symptoms of neutropenia include the following:

- Sore throat, mouth
- Low-grade fever
- Gingival pain and swelling
- Skin abscess
- Recurrent sinusitis, otitis
- Cough
- Shortness of breath
- Nasal congestion
- Diarrhea or loose stools
- Burning during urination
- Perirectal pain
- Unusual redness

Diagnostic Tests

- Blood cultures
- CBC with manual differential
- Antinuclear antibody (ANA)
- Rheumatoid factor (RF)
- Vitamin B_{12} and folate levels
- Basic metabolic panel (BMP)
- Kidney and liver function tests
- Urinalysis and urine culture
- Site-specific cultures such as stool, skin, sputum, and vascular access devices
- Skin biopsy, if new erythematous tender skin lesions are present
- HIV testing if risk factors are present
- Chest x-ray; ultrasound to rule out splenomegaly
- Bone marrow aspiration and biopsy may be indicated

HEMA/
ONCO

HEMA/ONCO

Management

■ Begin treatment with broad-spectrum antibiotics within 1 hr of obtaining cultures until an organism is identified.
■ Consider cefepime, meropenem, imipenem-cilastin, or piperacillin-tazobactam. Other agents may be used to manage complications, e.g., MRSA, VRE, ESBL, KPC.
■ Consider amphotericin B, a broad-spectrum azole, or an echinocandin if fever does not respond within 4–5 days or recurs.
■ Check temperature every 4 hr; avoid rectal temps.
■ Monitor for signs of infection.
■ Assess and monitor CBC with differential.
■ Discontinue any medications that could be the cause.
■ Use good skin care for wound and abrasions.
■ Educate patient's family members to avoid visiting if they have cold or flu-like symptoms.
■ Maintain good hand washing procedures. The National Comprehensive Cancer Network (NCCN) provided specific guidelines for oncology patients. Refer to https://www.nccn.org

Coagulopathy

Abnormalities in blood coagulation may comprise a large number of disorders, including deficiency (or single-factor) abnormalities and acquired forms associated with multiple coagulation abnormalities. The disorders are discussed here.

Vitamin K Deficiency

Vitamin K deficiency occurs when stores of this vitamin are deficient or abnormal, causing inhibition of normal coagulation.

Pathophysiology

■ Prothrombin factors VII, IX, and X (FVII, FIX, and FX) and proteins C and S are synthesized by the liver through a process that depends on vitamin K.
■ Vitamin K deficiency → synthesized hypofunctional by-products → inhibition of normal coagulation. These by-products do not bind to cellular phospholipid surfaces and therefore do not participate in cell-associated coagulation reactions. Coumadin produces a similar coagulation abnormality that antagonizes the action of vitamin K.
■ Because vitamin K is fat soluble, the absorption from the GI tract is decreased in biliary obstruction and in fat malabsorption syndromes.
■ Antibiotics that inhibit gut flora decrease the amount of vitamin K ordinarily supplied by these organisms.

Clinical Presentation
- Epistaxis, GI bleeding, menorrhagia, hematuria, and/or bleeding from puncture sites or invasive lines, wounds
- Prolonged PT and elevated INR

Diagnostic Tests
- PT (most sensitive early indicator)

Management
- Administer FFP (treatment of choice for acute hemorrhage or to reverse for a procedure).
- Administer vitamin K (1–10 mg × 3 days).
- Avoid drugs with hepatotoxicity.
- Continue to monitor PT.
- Assess for bleeding.
- Provide emotional support to patient and family.

Liver Disease
Coagulation disorder caused by liver disease is multifactorial and involves ↓ synthesis of coagulation proteins, ↑ clearance of FDPs, and ↑ fibrinolysis.

Pathophysiology
- In cirrhosis, FVII and protein C are the first to fall → a low FVII level, resulting in a prolonged PT. The remaining vitamin K–dependent factors decrease → prolonged aPTT. The fibrinogen level is usually maintained until end-stage disease. Because of impaired synthetic function → factors and fibrinogen may be functionally abnormal.
- In acute toxic or infectious hepatitis, impairment of coagulation correlates with the severity of cell damage.

Unlike the situation with other types of coagulopathy → coagulation factors and fibrinogen may be dysfunctional → because of abnormal hepatic synthetic function platelets may be dysfunctional by circulating FDPs that the liver fails to clear.

Clinical Presentation
- Bleeding
- Prolonged PT, activated PTT (aPTT)
- Elevated FDPs
- Low platelet count

Diagnostic Tests
- PT/PTT
- D-dimer assay
- Fibrin degradation/split products
- CBC
- Liver function tests

HEMA/ONCO

Management
- Administer blood products: FFP, platelets, and packed red blood cells.
- Avoid drugs with known hepatotoxicity.

Massive Transfusion

Coagulopathy can be caused by massive transfusion when the replacement of 1 or more blood volumes occurs in a 24-hr period (1 blood volume in a 70-kg adult is about a 5-L blood loss or transfusion volume of 10 units of packed red blood cells [PRBCs]). Common complications of massive transfusion are dilutional coagulopathy, DIC and fibrinolysis, hypothermia, citrate toxicity, hypokalemia, hyperkalemia, and infection.

Pathophysiology

Dilutional thrombocytopenia is the most common cause of bleeding after massive transfusion. If ongoing blood loss is replaced with only PRBCs → ↓ in platelet count → splenic pool mobilizing and counteracting loss during hemorrhage. If patient's count was high prior to transfusion → remainder may be adequate to prevent bleeding. If pretransfusion count was low or normal → the count may be 50,000–100,000/mcL → bleeding. Repletion of platelets → enhanced function of the coagulation factors and platelet plug formation. Platelets provide the surface on which many of the factors are activated and fibrin strands are formed.

Clinical Presentation
- Bleeding from areas other than the area of hemorrhage
- Low platelet count
- Prolonged PT, aPTT, and thrombin time
- Decreased fibrinogen

Diagnostic Tests
- PT/PTT
- CBC
- D-dimer assay
- Fibrin degradation/split products

Management
- Administer platelets.
- Administer cryoprecipitate.
- Replace electrolytes as needed.
- Provide support to patient and family members.

Refer to previous sections on DIC and HIT.

Oncological Emergencies

Oncological emergencies are complications or conditions of cancer and/or its treatments that require urgent or emergency interventions to avoid life-threatening situations.

Sepsis

Sepsis is a condition in which organisms enter into the bloodstream and cause activation of the host inflammation defense mechanism → release of cytokines and the activation of plasma protein cascade systems → septic shock → multisystem organ failure. Patients with cancer are at an ↑ risk for sepsis because of ↓ WBC and poor immune systems. Refer to the Multisystem Tab.

Disseminated Intravascular Coagulation (DIC)

See DIC as previously discussed.

Syndrome of Inappropriate Antidiuretic Hormone (SIADH)

SIADH is caused by malignant tumors, usually small cell lung cancer, tumors of the head and neck, tumors of the pancreas, and urological and gastric malignancies, that produce or secrete ADH or tumors that stimulate the brain to make and secrete ADH. SIADH can also be caused by medications frequently used by patients with cancer (e.g., morphine, cyclophosphamide) and by chemotherapy agents such as cisplatin, cyclophosphamide, imatinib, vinorelbine, alemtuzumab, ifosfamide, vincristine, and morphine. In SIADH, an excessive amount of water is reabsorbed by the kidney → ↑ in excessive fluid in circulation → hyponatremia and fluid retention.

Thoracic or mediastinal tumors can cause compression of major blood vessels → ↓ → ↓ fluid volume stimulation of the brain to secrete ADH, which can lead to ↓ urinary output.

The clinical presentation, diagnostic tests, and management of SIADH are discussed in the Endocrine Tab.

Management
■ Radiation or chemotherapy may be given to ↓ tumor progression and cause SIADH to subside and a return to normal ADH production.

Malignant Spinal Cord Compression

Compression of the spinal cord is caused by a tumor that directly enters the spinal cord or by vertebrae collapsing in response to deterioration of the bone secondary to a tumor. The compression site can be from a primary tumor, but compression usually results from metastases from the lung, prostate, breast, colon, thoracic spine, or pelvic lumbosacral spine.

Clinical Presentation

- Back pain
- Numbness
- Tingling
- Loss of urethral, vaginal, and rectal sensation
- Muscle weakness (neurological deficits are later signs)
- Paralysis (usually permanent)

Diagnostic Tests

- CT scan of torso
- MRI of spine

Management

- Provide early recognition and treatment.
- Perform comprehensive neurological examination.
- Administer high-dose corticosteroids to reduce swelling and relieve signs symptoms.
- Administer high-dose radiation to reduce tumor size and relieve symptoms.
- Be aware surgery may be indicated to remove the tumor.
- Apply external neck or back braces.

Malignant Hypercalcemia

Cancer in the bone releasing Ca^{2+} into bloodstream → ↑ serum Ca^{2+} levels. Cancer in other parts of the body (especially squamous cell tumors of the lung, head and neck, kidney, breast, or lymph nodes) → secretion of parathyroid hormone by the tumor → release of Ca^{2+} by the bone → ↑ serum Ca^{2+} levels. Decreased mobility and dehydration worsen hypercalcemia. Hypercalcemic crisis is usually defined as serum $Ca^{2+} > 14$ mg/dL (8.7–10.4 mg/dL normal) with acute signs and symptoms.

Clinical Presentation

The mnemonic associated with this diagnosis: "Bones, stones, moans, and groans"

- Fatigue, weakness, lethargy, or depression
- Loss of appetite
- Nausea and vomiting

- Paralytic ileus
- Constipation
- Polyuria (early sign)
- Kidney stones
- Severe muscle weakness
- Loss of deep-tendon reflexes
- More severe changes: dehydration, ECG changes (shortened QT interval)
- CNS changes including headache or confusion
- Seizures
- Coma

Diagnostic Tests
- Parathyroid hormone levels.
- BMP every 6 hr.
- Ca^{2+} levels. Hypercalcemia may produce ECG changes such as shortened QT or prolonged PR.
- CT, MRI, or ultrasound may be indicated to assess parathyroid disease or tumor.

Management
- Provide oral hydration.
- Provide IV hydration with normal saline. Prevent volume overload.
- Administer medications to decrease Ca^{2+} levels temporarily.
- Administer glucocorticoids: prednisone or hydrocortisone.
- Administer calcitonin Miacalcin or galliSheum nitrate (Ganite).
- Administer bisphosphonates: pamidronate (Aredia), etidronate (Didronel), zoledronic acid (Zometa).
- Consider IV phosphate and cinacalcet (Sensipar). Consider furosemide (Lasix) to increase calcium excretion. Avoid thiazide diuretics.
- Dialysis may be indicated to decrease serum Ca^{2+} levels in life-threatening situations or in patients with renal impairment.

Superior Vena Cava Syndrome (SVCS)

SVCS occurs when the SVC is compressed or obstructed by tumor growth → painful life-threatening emergency, most often seen in patients with thoracic malignant disease, especially adenocaricinoma associated with lung cancer. SVCS results in blockage of blood flow in the venous system of the chest, neck, and upper trunk. SVCS is also common in patients with intravascular devices and in hypercoagulability syndromes.

Clinical Presentation
Early Symptoms
- Dyspnea most common symptom. Edema of the face, especially around the eyes, when patient arises from night's sleep. Sensation of head fullness
- Dysphagia, cough, and hoarseness

HEMA/
ONCO

- Tightness of shirt or collar (Stokes' sign) as compression worsens
- New onset of back pain, worsening at night with lying down
- Epistaxis

Late Symptoms
- Chest pain or signs of decreased cardiac output → hypotension
- Hemorrhage
- Edema in arms and hands
- Venous distention of neck veins
- Dyspnea
- Pleural effusions
- Erythema of upper body
- Cyanosis
- Mental status changes
- Death (if compression not relieved)

Diagnostic Tests
- Spiral CT with contrast or MRI of chest
- Selective venography
- ECG

Management
- Monitor cardiac, respiratory, and neurological status.
- Keep head of bed elevated. Control nausea and vomiting.
- Maintain patent airway. Provide O_2 therapy as indicated.
- Administer diuretics, anticoagulants, and corticosteroids as needed.
- Provide high-dose radiation to the mediastinal area (provides temporary relief)
- Avoid chest and neck central venous catheters.
- Interventional radiology may place a metal stent in the vena cava to relieve swelling
- Be aware thrombolytic therapy or follow-up angioplasty may be needed to keep the stent open longer.
- Surgery rarely is performed. The tumor may have caused a large increase in intrathoracic pressure, so closing the chest postoperatively would be impossible. Surgery may be indicated in patients who have a life expectancy of >3 mo and are at risk for paraplegia.
- Know best treatment results occur in the early stages of SVCS.
- Monitor for complications such as right-sided heart failure, blood vessel rupture, and radiation pneumonitis.

Tumor Lysis Syndrome (TLS)

Tumor lysis syndrome (TLS) occurs when large numbers of tumor cells are destroyed rapidly ← the release of intracellular contents (K^+ and purines) into the bloodstream faster than the body can eliminate them → tissue damage and death if severe or untreated → ↑ K^+ levels → severe hyperkalemia → severe cardiac dysfunction. An ↑ in purines (converted in the liver to uric acid) released into bloodstream → hyperuricemia → precipitation of these crystals in the kidney → sludge in the tubules → blockage → acute renal failure. TLS is most often seen in patients receiving chemotherapy or radiation for cancers highly responsive to this treatment, including leukemia (acute lymphocytic leukemia, acute myelogenous leukemia), lymphoma (non-Hodgkin's lymphoma, Burkitt's lymphoma), small cell lung carcinoma, germ cell tumors, inflammatory breast cancer, melanoma, and multiple myeloma. This oncological emergency is a positive sign the treatment is working.

Clinical Presentation

TLS is diagnosed if one or more of these three conditions arise:

- Cardiac arrhythmias
- Arthralgias from gout flare-up
- Signs and symptoms of increased phosphorus, K^+, Ca^{2+}, and uric acid

Diagnostic Tests

- CMP including uric acid level
- CBC
- Urinary uric acid/creatinine ratio
- ECG. Changes caused by K^+ and calcium abnormalities
- CT or ultrasound of mediastinal areas, abdomen, or retroperitoneum

Management

- Monitor fluid and electrolyte balance including intake and output; osmolarity.
- Provide IV hydration, which ↓ serum K^+ level and ↑ kidney filtration rate.
- Instruct patient to drink at least 3–5 L of fluid the day before, the day of, and 3 days after treatment (especially in patients with tumors highly sensitive to treatment, as mentioned earlier).
- Ensure that some fluids are alkaline (Na^+).
- ECG monitoring to detect arrhythmias.
- Health teach importance of consistent fluid intake over 24 hr (help patient draw up a schedule).
- Health teach importance of taking antiemetics after treatment to prevent nausea and vomiting, which would hinder fluid intake.
- Administer diuretics, especially osmotic types, to increase urine flow. Use with caution because diuretics may cause dehydration.
- Administer medications that increase secretion of purines: allopurinol (Zyloprim), rasburicase (Elitek).
- Administer medications to decrease hyperkalemia: sodium polystyrene sulfonate (Kayexalate), either orally or rectally by enema.
- Administer IV infusion containing dextrose and insulin if hyperglycemic.
- Initiate hemodialysis or CRRT as needed.

HEMA/
ONCO

Leukemia

Leukemia is the uncontrolled neoplastic reproduction of WBCs. Causes include significant bone marrow damage that can result from radiation, drugs, or chemicals. Genetic, viral, and environmental factors also play a role in developing leukemia.

Pathophysiology

Myeloid Leukemia

- **Acute:** Malignant alterations in hematopoietic stem cells. Risk factors include advanced age, therapeutic radiation, receipt of supportive care, smoking, and exposure to chemicals. It is the most common form of myeloid leukemia among adults.

- **Chronic:** Uncontrolled mutation of myeloid cells. This disease is rare in children, and risk increases with age. The incidence of this type of leukemia is increased with radiation exposure.

Lymphocytic Leukemia

- **Acute:** Large numbers of bone marrow stem cells develop into lymphocytes. Most prevalent in children 3–7 yr old (most common childhood acute leukemia).

- **Chronic:** Only leukemia not related to radiation or chemicals. B lymphocytes do not go through apoptosis ← excessive cells in bone marrow and blood ⟩ enlarged nodes → hepatomegaly and splenomegaly ← anemia and thrombocytopenia. This type of leukemia has a slight genetic predisposition.

Clinical Presentation

Acute Myeloid Leukemia

- Fatigue
- Shortness of breath or dyspnea on exertion
- Bruising or bleeding, especially from lungs, GI, and CNS
- Petechiae rash
- Weight loss or anorexia
- Fever
- Infection
- Pain from enlargement of liver and spleen
- Gum hyperplasia or bleeding gums
- Bone pain
- Anginal chest pain or MI may be first sign of acute leukemia

Chronic Myeloid Leukemia

- Many patients asymptomatic for long periods of time
- Malaise
- Loss of appetite
- Weight loss
- Spleen tenderness and enlargement

Acute Lymphocytic Leukemia
- Reduced leukocytes, erythrocytes, and platelets
- Bone and joint pain
- Easy bruising and bleeding (gums, skin, nose, abnormal periods)
- Feeling weak or tired
- Fever
- Loss of appetite and weight loss
- Paleness
- Pain or feeling of fullness below ribs
- Abdominal swelling or left upper quadrant fullness; feeling full after eating small amounts
- Petechiae rash
- Lymphadenopathy (neck, axilla, groin)
- Night sweats
- Pain from enlarged liver, or spleen
- Headache
- Vomiting

Chronic Lymphocytic Leukemia
- Asymptomatic in many cases
- Elevated WBCs
- Enlarged lymph nodes and spleen
- Possible development of B-symptoms: fever, night sweats, weight loss, bacterial infections, and viral infections

Diagnostic Tests
- CBC with differential
- Coagulation studies: PT, fibrinogen, fibrin split products
- Peripheral blood smear. Blood chemistries and blood cultures if indicated
- Bone marrow aspiration and biopsy
- Lumbar puncture (to check for leukemia cells in spinal fluid)
- Immunophenotyping
- CT, CXR, MUGA scanning, and ECG may be helpful

Management
- Perform daily assessment of body systems. Look for signs of DIC.
- Monitor for anemia and infections.
- Consider platelet transfusions, FFP, or cryoprecipitate.
- Administer chemotherapy and assess for side effects.
- Assess for side effects of radiation therapy.
- Monitor CBC closely.
- Maintain bleeding precautions.
- Provide nutritional support.
- Provide meticulous oral hygiene.
- Provide perirectal hygiene.

- Apply mask to patient when out of room.
- Assess patient's anxiety level.
- Monitor intake and output, and assess hydration status.
- Administer analgesic and antipyretics; provide comfort measures as needed.
- Provide emotional support to patient and family members.

Bone Marrow Transplantation

Bone marrow transplantation is the aspiration of marrow from the posterior iliac crest of a marrow donor with the use of regional or general anesthesia and the IV transfusion of the marrow into a donor-matched recipient. The three kinds of bone marrow transplants are autologous bone marrow transplant (patient's own), allogeneic bone marrow transplant (from a donor), and umbilical cord blood transplant (stem cells from a newborn baby's umbilical cord immediately after birth).

Procedure

Before being ready to receive the transplant, the patient must:

- Undergo high-dose chemotherapy, radiation, or both (myeloablative treatment) or lower doses of chemotherapy and radiation (nonmyeloablative) in an effort to treat the underlying disease and overcome rejection.
- Be treated with immunosuppressive drugs to decrease the risk of rejection. T factors influencing the outcome of bone marrow transplantation include:
  - Disease status at transplantation
  - Type of donor
  - Recipient's age
  - Comorbid medical conditions

Early-Stage Complications

The time of greatest risk is between 0 and 100 days.

- Rejection
- Mucositis, pain issues secondary to oral ulcerations and reactive herpes virus; oral nutritional deficits secondary to oral pain
- Hemorrhage, caused by chronic thrombocytopenia and tissue injury; can be life threatening, but rare
- Common minor bleeding, such as petechiae, epistaxis, or GI or GU bleeding (not life-threatening, but worrisome to patients)
- Infections
  - Bacterial; usually gram-positive, but can be gram-negative
  - Fungal
  - Viral; can be life-threatening to these patients

- Acute graft-versus-host disease: One of the most serious and challenging complications; caused by immunologically competent donor-derived T cells that react with recipient tissue antigens
- Veno-occlusive disease of the liver: One of the most feared complications; signs and symptoms include unexplained weight gain, jaundice, abdominal pain, and ascites
- Pulmonary complications: A common problem; causes of lung injury or pneumonitis can be infection, chemical, bleeding, or idiopathic

Management

- Provide emotional support to patient and family.
- Perform good hand washing and aseptic technique.
- Use reverse isolation procedures.
- Monitor CBC and BMP laboratory tests frequently.
- Provide frequent oral care.
- Assess for signs and symptoms of bleeding.
- Monitor vital signs every 4 hr or more frequently if needed.
- Administer immunosuppressive drugs as ordered.
- Consider IV or enteral nutritional support.

Coagulation

Lab	Conventional	SI Units
Activated coagulation time (ACT)	90–130 sec	90–130 sec
Activated partial thromboplastin time (aPTT) (>70 sec)	25–39 sec	25–39 sec
Bleeding time (>14 min)	2–7 min	2–7 min
Fibrinogen (<80 mg/dL)	200–400 mg/dL	2–4 g/L
International normalized ratio (INR) (>5)	Normal: <2 Target therapeutic: 2–3	<2 2–3
Plasminogen	80%–120% of normal	80%–120% of normal
Platelets (<20,000; >1,000,000)	150,000–450,000/mm^3	150–450 109/L
Prothrombin time (PT) (>27 sec)	10–13 sec	10–13 sec
Thrombin time	11–15 sec	11–15 sec

Glucose Control in the Critically Ill Patient

Hyperglycemia in hospitalized patients has been linked to poorer outcomes:

- Increased length of stay, morbidity, and mortality
- Development of DKA, HHS, and ketosis
- Osmotic diuresis causing electrolyte abnormalities, volume depletion, and dehydration
- Impaired leukocyte function leading to impaired wound healing and increased risk of infection; greater antibiotic usage

Conditions that trigger hyperglycemia include:

- Pancreatitis and other pancreatic and endocrine disorders
- Sepsis
- Pregnancy
- Head injury
- Glucocorticoid therapy
- Immunosuppressants (e.g., tacrolimus, cyclosporine); immune dysfunction
- Sympathomimetic agents (e.g., norepinephrine, dopamine, dobutamine, isoproterenol)
- Enteral and parenteral nutrition
- Liver or renal failure; peritoneal dialysis
- Stress-induced insulin resistance or a hypermetabolic stress state; surgery
- Dextrose containing IV infusions

Management

- The American Diabetes Association (ADA) and the American Association of Clinical Endocrinologists (AACE) now recommend the following serum glucose targets for critically ill patients:
  - Serum glucose of 140–180 mg/dL is recommended.
  - Serum glucose of 110–140 mg/dL is acceptable in selected patients but increases the risk of hypoglycemia.
- Tight glucose control remains controversial.
- For non-critically ill patients, the preprandial serum glucose target is <140 mg/dL and the random serum glucose target is <180 mg/dL. In older patients, the serum glucose target is 140–180 mg/dL. These may be considered target levels for transfer out of an ICU.
- Insulin should not be started unless the patient exhibits persistent hyperglycemia (serum glucose >180 mg/dL).
- Scheduled basal and meal insulin is recommended to improve glycemic control compared with sliding-scale insulin coverage alone. Subcutaneous insulin may be administered every 6 hr.
- IV infusion of insulin is preferred to subcutaneous insulin administration.

- Blood glucose measurement accuracy may be affected by anemia; hypoperfusion states; drugs such as levodopa, dopamine, and mannitol; high uric acid levels; and high unconjugated bilirubin, among others.

CAUTION: Hypoglycemia among critically ill patients increases the risk of death. There should be a well-devised plan for transitioning the patient from an IV insulin infusion to subcutaneous insulin.

- IV insulin infusion protocols and algorithms differ by hospitals. Examples include:
  - The Portland protocol:
    - https://oregon.providence.org/~/media/Files/Providence%20OR%20PDF/ Protocol_150200_FLOOR.pdf
  - Yale University protocol:
    - http://inpatient.aace.com/sites/all/files/Yale_IIP_MICU120-160_2011.pdf
  - University of Washington algorithm:
    - http://www.scoap.org/downloads/Insulin-Orders-Related-to-Perioperative -Care-and-Handoffs.pdf
  - Computer-based systems: Glucommander and eGlycemic Management System, GlucoStabilizer, proportional integral derivative algorithm

Institution-specific care:

_____

_____

_____

_____

_____

Diabetic Ketoacidosis (DKA)

DKA is a life-threatening metabolic complication caused by an absence or inadequate amount of insulin. Affecting those mostly with type 1 diabetes but not uncommon in type 2 diabetes, it is marked by three concurrent abnormalities: severe hyperglycemia (300–1,000 dL), dehydration, and electrolyte loss (ketonemia, ketonuria, and metabolic acidosis [bicarbonate level <15 mEq/L and pH <7.30]).

Pathophysiology

DKA can be initiated by trauma or conditions such as new-onset diabetes, heart failure, pancreatitis, infection, illness, surgery, or stress. The most common causes are infections including urinary tract infections and pneumonia. The body under stress $\rightarrow \downarrow$ in the amount of insulin $\rightarrow \downarrow$ of glucose entering cells and $\uparrow$ glucose production by the liver $\rightarrow$ hyperglycemia $\rightarrow$ liver attempting to remove excess glucose by excreting glucose with water, Na^+, and $K^+ \rightarrow$ polyuria $\rightarrow$ dehydration.

DKA can also be caused by a lack of insulin ↓ ↑ fatty acid and glycerol ↓ fatty acids converted into ketones → metabolic acidosis ↓ ↑ respiratory rate and abdominal pain, and acetone breath. Can lead to hyperkalemia, hypoxemia, coma, and death. For every 0.1 change in pH → change in K⁺.

Clinical Presentation

- Severe hyperglycemia
- Polyuria and polydipsia are the most common early symptoms.
- Dry mucous membranes, thirst, loss of skin turgor, dehydration
- Weakness, malaise, fatigability
- Headache
- Ketonic (acetone) or fruity breath
- Anorexia, nausea and vomiting, diarrhea, weight loss
- Abdominal pain or cramps, usually generalized or epigastric
- Rigid abdomen, irregular bowel sounds
- Tachypnea or Kussmaul's respirations
- Hypothermia, decreased perspiration
- Hypotension and tachycardia; shock
- Glycosuria
- Ketones in blood and urine
- Metabolic acidosis: pH <7.3, bicarbonate <15 mmol/L, blood glucose >14 mmol/L, ketonuria
- Lethargy mild disorientation or confusion. May progress to stupor and coma

Diagnostic Tests

- ECG if comorbidities suspected
- Chest x-ray
- Urinalysis (note presence of ketones)
- CBC
- Serum electrolytes and chemistries, glucose and ketone levels, BUN, and creatinine
- Urine, sputum, and wound and blood cultures if infection suspected
- ABGs and ↑ anion gap (8–16 mEq/L or 8–16 mmol/L normal). Bicarbonate levels
- Serum osmolarity (↑)
- Cardiac enzymes
- Amylase and lipase levels
- Serum or capillary beta-hydroxybutyrate levels

NOTE: Serum and urine should be negative for ketones. High serum glucose levels → osmotic diuresis → dilutional hyponatremia and hypokalemia and dehydration.

Management

- Administer O_2. Provide airway support. Monitor ABGs or Svo_2.
- Monitor respiratory rate and rhythm and blood pH. Sodium bicarbonate administration is controversial. If indicated, infuse 100–150 mL of 1.4% concentration. Repeat every half hour. May worsen hypokalemia.
- Monitor vital signs. Administer vasopressors as indicated. Assess for arrhythmias.
- Assess for changes in mental status.
- Assess for signs of hypokalemia. Replace K^+ as needed.
- Monitor serum glucose and ketone levels every 1–2 hr until patient stable → every 4–6 hr.
- Monitor serum or capillary beta-hydroxybutyrate levels to assess effectiveness of DKA treatment.
- Provide insulin replacement (insulin drip) as per policy. Use only short-acting insulin to correct hyperglycemia with an optimum glucose decline of 100 mg/dL/hr.
- Provide electrolyte replacement.
- Provide aggressive fluid resuscitation and monitor intake and output. Most patients require rapid infusion of 500 mL 0.9% NS or LR over 10–15 min. if systolic BP less than 90 mm Hg or 1,000 mL over 60 min. for systolic BP greater than 90 mm Hg. Continue with 1,000 mL/hr during second hour, 1,000 mL during the following 2 hr and then 1,000 mL every 4 hr dependent on degree of dehydration and hemodynamic parameters. Administer 5%–10% D/0.45% NS when blood sugar decreases to less than 180 mg/dL. After initial stabilization, administer 0.45% NS at 200–1,000 mL/hr to match losses due to osmotic diuresis.
- Monitor for Somogyi effect (rebound hyperglycemia after an episode of hypoglycemia).
- Provide seizure and safety precautions.

Hyperosmolar Hyperglycemic State (HHS)

Previously called hyperosmolar hyperglycemic nonketotic coma (HHNC), HHS is an acute hyperglycemic crisis that usually occurs in patients with type 2 diabetes mellitus who develop a concomitant illness leading to reduced fluid intake, infection (pneumonia, UTI, sepsis), or noncompliance with diabetic regimen.

Pathophysiology

Insulin deficiency → hyperosmolarity → cell dehydration and hyperglycemia → osmotic diuresis. May progress to coma.

ENDO

Clinical Presentation

- Extreme hyperglycemia with serum glucose ≥600 mg/dL
- Serum hyperosmolarity of ≥320 mOsm/kg
- Severe dehydration; an average of 9 L not uncommon
- Poor skin turgor, sunken eyes, dry mouth
- Tachycardia, hypotension
- Visual changes or disturbances, sensory deficits
- Polyuria, polydipsia
- No significant ketoacidosis. Serum pH usually >7.30 and bicarbonate concentration >15 mEq/L
- Hypotension, tachycardia, tachypnea
- Hypothermia a poor prognostic factor in HHS
- Fatigue, drowsiness, lethargy, stupor, delirium
- Neurological changes suggestive of CVA or other neurological conditions
- Seizures and coma

Diagnostic Tests

- Serum electrolytes and chemistries including BUN and creatinine
- CBC
- Serum and urine osmolarity and ketones. Mild-moderate ketosis may be present
- Urinalysis
- Urine, sputum, and blood cultures if infection suspected
- ECG. MI and pulmonary embolism can precipitate HHS. ECG changes due to electrolyte disturbances
- ABGs to assess acidosis
- Chest x-ray if pneumonia or other comorbidities suspected
- If neurological symptoms present or cerebral edema suspected, head CT

Management

- Correct fluid and electrolyte imbalances. Administer 500 mL bolus of isotonic (0.9%) NS IV followed by 1–2 L of either 0.9% or 0.45% NS in the first 2 hr. Use 0.45% NS once BP and urine output adequate. Administer all IV fluids cautiously or at a slower rate if cardiac or renal disease present and to prevent cerebral edema.
- Monitor blood glucose levels carefully. Consider hourly testing during first 24–48 hr of treatment.
- Insulin infusion as per policy. Blood glucose levels sensitive to insulin because the patient may still be secreting some insulin.

- Monitor serum osmolarity or osmolality. Serum osmolarity = $(2 \times Na) +$ $(glucose/18) + (BUN/2.8)$. Normal value = 280–290 mOsm/kg. Higher values correlate with level of impaired LOC.
- Assess VS, hemodynamic parameters, intake and output.
- Assess hydration status frequently. Monitor electrolytes when osmotic diuresis occurs, especially Na^+ and K^+.
- Assess respiratory and neurological status. Hypoglycemia and decompensated hyperglycemia may manifest as mental changes.
- No evidence to support the use of sodium bicarbonate. Consider if pH <7.0.
- Provide ventilatory support as indicated.
- Provide seizure and safety precautions.

Diabetes Insipidus (DI)

DI has been defined as the excretion of a large volume (>3L/24 hr) of dilute urine (<300m Osm/kg) caused by a decrease in secretion of vasopressin (ADH) or resistance of kidneys to vasopressin.

Pathophysiology

Decrease ADH → decreased ability of kidneys to reabsorb water → increase in urine output or excessive urination (polyuria and nocturia) → excretion of large amounts of dilute urine → hyponatremia → excessive thirst (polydipsia). Can also lead to dehydration and decreased cardiac output → decreased BP → hypovolemic shock.

Types of DI include:

- Central DI, which includes neurogenic
  - No ADH or inadequate synthesis or secretion of ADH
  - Cause can be congenital or idiopathic:
    - CNS tumors
    - Cerebrovascular disease, aneurysms, thrombosis, or trauma
    - Infection
    - Granulomas
    - Pregnancy
    - Brain death
- Nephrogenic DI: rare genetic disorder
  - Secretion of ADH but no stimulation to the nephron's collecting tubules
  - Cause can be congenital or idiopathic:
    - Obstruction that hinders normal urine excretion
    - Chronic tubulointerstitial disease, pyelonephritis, polycystic disease
    - Medications
    - Electrolyte imbalance

- Dipsogenic DI
  - Caused by a defect or damage to the thirst mechanism in the hypothalamus
  - Results in an abnormal increase in thirst with an increased fluid intake that suppresses ADH secretion and increases urine output
- Gestational DI
  - Occurs only during pregnancy

Clinical Presentation

- Symptoms may be transient, temporary, partial, or permanent
- Polyuria or large volume (3–20 L) of very diluted urine with a low specific gravity (1.001–1.005) (volume does not decrease even with restricted fluids)
- Polydipsia or extreme thirst, especially for cold water and sometimes ice or ice water
- Nocturia
- Dehydration
- Weight loss, dizziness, weakness and fatigue, sleep disturbances
- Drowsiness, confusion, and headache may indicate water intoxication
- Symptoms of hypovolemic shock: changes in level of consciousness (LOC), tachycardia, tachypnea, and hypotension

Diagnostic Tests

- Water deprivation test (Miller-Moses test)
- AVP (desmopressin) stimulation test, 3% hypertonic saline infusion test
- Plasma ADH
- Plasma and urine osmolarity
- Serum chemistries and electrolytes
- Urinalysis including specific gravity
- Brain or pituitary MRI or CT scan

Management

- Management of DI is highly dependent on the type.
- Administer desmopressin (DDAVP, Stimate) for central DI; ineffective in nephrogenic DI.
- Administer synthetic vasopressin (Pitressin).
- Administer chlorpropamide (Novo-Propamide).
- Administer hydrochlorothiazide (Microzide), amiloride (Midamor), diclofenac (Voltaren) or ketoprofen (Frotek) for nephrogenic DI.
- Consider indomethacin (Indocin), or NSAIDs (ibuprofen or naproxen).
- Monitor vital signs frequently.
- Assess neurological status for changes in mentation.

- Monitor and treat fluid and electrolyte balance. Infuse fluids at a rate of <500–750 mL/hr.
- Assess intake and output. Weigh daily. Monitor for fluid retention.
- Administer hypotonic IV fluids to match urine output. Monitor urine specific gravity.
- Assess for water intoxication: drowsiness, lightheadedness, headache → seizures and coma.
- If surgery is indicated, provide emotional support to patient and family.

Adrenal Crisis—Acute Adrenal Insufficiency

Acute adrenal crisis, also known as acute adrenal insufficiency, is a serious complication of a dysfunctional adrenal gland causing difficulties in producing aldosterone and cortisol hormones. May also be caused by adrenal hemorrhage.

Pathophysiology

Destruction of adrenal cortex → hindered secretion of aldosterone and cortisol → Addison's disease → hypoglycemia and hypovolemic shock → coma and death.
   Risk factors for adrenal crisis include:

- Recently rapid discontinued long-term corticosteroid therapy
- Injury to or infection of the adrenal gland
- Chronic adrenal insufficiency
- Bilateral adrenalectomy
- Medications that suppress adrenal hormones
- Medications that enhance steroid metabolism
- Sepsis and septic shock

Clinical Presentation

- Serious muscle weakness, fatigue
- Hyperthermia or hypothermia
- Hyperpigmentation
- Hypoglycemia
- Fever
- Headache
- Nausea, vomiting, poor appetite or anorexia
- Dehydration and electrolyte imbalances
- Abdominal or flank pain
- Diarrhea
- Altered mental status, lethargy, or confusion

- Hypotension, circulatory shock
- Tachycardia, dysrhythmias
- Lack of response to vasopressors

Diagnostic Tests

- Cosyntropin (ACTH) stimulation test
- Plasma cortisol
- Metyrapone (Metopirone) test for diagnosis
- CBC, serum electrolytes and chemistries, BUN and creatinine
- Serum thyroid levels
- Urine, sputum, and blood cultures if infection suspected
- CT scan or ultrasound of the adrenal glands
- CXR may be indicated
- ECG for prolongation of QT interval

Management

- Assess vital signs and hemodynamic parameters as indicated. Consider vasopressors.
- Assess respiratory status and oxygenation.
- Assess for arrhythmias.
- Weigh daily.
- Strictly monitor intake and output and renal function. Correct hypovolemia.
- Monitor serum electrolytes and glucose levels frequently.
- Administer cortisol replacement medications (hydrocortisone IV).
- Insert nasogastric tube if vomiting.
- Reorient and minimize stress.
- Provide small, frequent meals and nutritional supplements.
- Administer aggressive fluid and electrolyte therapy.

CAUTION: Patients with Addison's disease should not receive insulin because of resultant hypoglycemia.

Thyroid Storm—Thyrotoxic Crisis—Thyrotoxicosis

Thyroid storm is a rare, life-threatening complication of a severe form of hyperthyroidism that is characterized by high fever, extreme tachycardia, and altered mental status. It is precipitated by stress and usually has an abrupt onset. Also called thyrotoxic crisis or thyrotoxicosis.

Pathophysiology

Thyrotropin-releasing hormone (TRH) is released from the hypothalamus after exposure to stress → the pituitary gland releasing thyroid-stimulating hormone (TSH) → causes the release of thyroid hormone (T_3 and T_4) from the thyroid gland → T_3 active form of thyroid hormone → increased levels of thyroid hormone leading to hyperthyroidism or thyrotoxicosis → if precipitated by stress (surgery, infection, trauma, DKA, heart failure, pulmonary embolism, toxemia of pregnancy, thyroid hormone ingestion, radioiodine therapy, discontinuation of antithyroid), further increase in serum thyroid hormone → thyroid storm. Can lead to vascular collapse, hypotension, coma, and death.

Clinical Presentation

- High fever, hyperthermia
- Heat intolerance, excessive sweating
- Severe tachycardia (>200 bpm), hypertension with heart failure and shock
- Cardiovascular dysfunction and arrhythmias possibly primary symptoms in elderly patients
- Goiter
- Vision disturbances, exophthalmos
- Nausea, vomiting
- Restlessness, agitation, irritability
- Tremors, muscle weakness
- Severe agitation, confusion, delirium, psychosis, stupor, weakness, somnolence
- Seizures, coma

Exaggerated symptoms of hyperthyroidism with disturbances of major systems:

- GI:
  - Weight loss
  - Diarrhea
  - Abdominal pain
  - Jaundice
- CV:
  - Edema
  - Hypertension with wide pulse pressure or hypotension with shock
  - Chest pain
  - Shortness of breath, dyspnea, cough
  - Palpitations
  - Cardiac arrhythmias, especially atrial fibrillation, supraventricular tachycardia, sinus bradycardia, heart block, ventricular dysrhythmias
  - Can progress to heart failure

ENDO

Diagnostic Tests

- Serum thyroid tests
- Liver function tests
- CBC, serum electrolytes, chemistries, especially calcium
- ABGs, ECG
- Thyroid scan
- CT, MRI

Management

"Triangle of treatment":

- Decrease sympathetic outflow (Administer beta blockers: esmolol [Brevibloc] the drug of choice. Consider propranolol [Inderal]. Calcium channel blockers may be administered if beta blockers contraindicated.)
- Decrease production of thyroid hormone (Administer propylthiouracil [PTU], methimazole [Tapazole], or radioactive iodine [Lugol's iodine or potassium iodide].) Monitor for severe liver injury or acute liver failure.
- Decrease peripheral conversion of T_4 to T_3 (PTU, beta blockers, and glucocorticoids such as hydrocortisone [Solu-Cortef] [preferred] or dexamethasone [Decadron]).
- Assess neurological, respiratory, and cardiovascular status.
- Monitor vital signs frequently.
- Provide cooling measures for fever. Give acetaminophen; salicylates are contraindicated.
- Monitor for cardiac arrhythmias and signs of heart failure and cardiac collapse.
- Monitor ABGs and provide continuous SvO_2 monitoring. Administer O_2 or ventilatory support as indicated.
- Monitor serum glucose levels closely.
- Administer IV fluids containing dextrose to replace liver glycogen.
- Correct electrolyte imbalances.
- Monitor intake and output.
- Maintain a quiet environment.
- Administer bile acid sequestrants.
- Plasmapheresis only as life-saving measure.

Syndrome of Inappropriate Antidiuretic Hormone (SIADH)

SIADH is the continuous secretion of ADH from the pituitary gland despite low osmolarity. It is frequently manifested by hyponatremia and water intoxication. Oat cell lung cancer is the most common cause of SIADH.

Pathophysiology

Malignant tumors, pulmonary and CNS disorders, and select medications → ↑ secretion of ADH → hyponatremia → ↑ water retention → stimulation of renin-angiotensin system → ↑ excretion of sodium in urine and excess of water.

Clinical Presentation

- Hyponatremia is characteristic feature of SIADH (serum Na^+ <135 mmol/L), along with serum hypo-osmolality
- Concentrated urine and decreased urine output
- Water retention and weight gain, edema despite low urine output
- Lethargy, weakness, fatigue, malaise
- Dilutional hyponatremia (serum Na^+ 115–120 mEq/L)
- Poor skin turgor, dry mucosa, thirst
- Headache
- Decreased saliva
- Orthostatic hypotension, tachycardia
- Loss of appetite, nausea, vomiting
- Abdominal or muscle cramps
- Extreme muscle weakness
- Irritability, confusion, disorientation, delirium, hallucinations
- Emotional and behavioral changes
- Seizures, coma, and death if serum Na^+ <110 mEq/L

Diagnostic Tests

- Comprehensive metabolic panel including BUN and creatinine. Serum uric acid
- CBC
- Radioimmunoassay for ADH/AVP and serum cortisol; thyroid-stimulating hormone
- Urinalysis and specific gravity
- Urine Na^+ and electrolytes

- Plasma and urine osmolarity
- Ultrasound of kidneys
- Chest x-ray and CT or MRI of head

Management

- Assess cardiac and respiratory status for heart failure.
- Monitor vital signs frequently; O_2 saturation, and arrhythmias.
- Assess for edema of extremities. Administer loop diuretics (e.g., furosemide [Lasix]) or osmotic agents (e.g., mannitol [Osmitrol]).
- Institute fluid restrictions to 500–1,000 mL/day.
- Monitor intake and output and fluid balance.
- Weigh daily.
- Increase Na+ intake.
- Administer 3% hypertonic saline cautiously if low serum Na+ levels.
- Closely monitor electrolytes, especially Na+ levels.
- Monitor for CNS changes.
- Administer demeclocycline (Declomycin, Ledermycin) to treat hyponatremia by inhibiting the action of ADH.
- Administer vasopressin-2 receptor antagonists such as conivaptan (Vaprisol) or tolvaptan (Samsca) to treat hyponatremia.
- Institute seizure and safety precautions.
- Radiation or chemotherapy may be administered to reduce tumor progression, with resulting normal ADH production.

Myxedema Coma or Crisis

Myxedema coma is a form of severe hypothyroidism that results in slowing of bodily metabolic processes. Symptoms can be manifested in all organ systems. It is usually precipitated by a secondary condition such as infection, a systemic disease, or select medications.

Pathophysiology

Hypothyroidism → ↓ metabolic rate, ↓ O_2 consumption → peripheral vasoconstriction → diastolic hypertension and ↑ blood volume.

Clinical Presentation

- Fatigue
- Hypothermia and cold intolerance; absence of shivering

- Absence of fever in the presence of infection
- Abdominal distention, goiter, decreased bowel sounds, constipation
- Dry skin, pallor, cold extremities
- Periorbital edema; sacral or peripheral edema
- Normal systolic BP, elevated diastolic BP, slow heart rate, depressed respirations
- Hypotension, shock
- Lethargy, weakness, confusion, paranoia, stupor, delirium
- Seizures, coma

Diagnostic Tests

- Serum thyroid tests
- Serum cortisol level
- Serum electrolytes and chemistries including BUN, creatinine, and lactate
- Serum osmolarity
- Serum CPK, AST, SCOT
- CBC
- Creatine kinase (CK) levels to rule out MI
- Urinalysis
- ABGs
- Electrocardiogram; echocardiogram if pericardial effusion suspected
- Chest x-ray, abdominal series, CT or MRI

Management

- Provide airway support. Monitor ABGs or pulse oximetry.
- Monitor cardiac and respiratory status.
- Monitor vital signs. Assess for arrhythmias. Hypotension may respond to crystalloid infusion or vasopressors. Consider hemodynamic monitoring.
- Assess for changes in mental status.
- Treat hypothermias by providing passive rewarming of patient with blankets and warm room. External warming is contraindicated.
- Correct fluid and electrolyte imbalances.
- Monitor and treat serum glucose levels.
- Administer levothyroxine (Synthroid, Levoxyl) IV.
- Consider steroids (Hydrocortisone IV) after a cortisol level is obtained.
- Avoid sedatives, barbiturates, narcotics, or any drugs that may be slowly metabolized, causing prolonged effects.
- Provide seizure and safety precautions.

Systemic Inflammatory Response Syndrome (SIRS)

SIRS is a widespread systemic inflammation that may be caused by either an infectious or a noninfectious process. It may progress to acute respiratory failure, acute renal failure, disseminated intravascular coagulopathy (DIC), sepsis, septic shock, multiple organ dysfunction syndrome (MODS), and eventually death.

SIRS is diagnosed if two or more of the following signs are present:

- Temp >38°C (100.4°F) or <36°C (96.8°F)
- HR >90 bpm
- Tachypnea with RR >20 bpm or $Paco_2$ <32 mm Hg
- WBC count >12,000 cells/mm³ or <4,000 cells/mm³, or >10% immature bands

Very young and very old patients may not present with typical symptoms. Tachycardia may not be evident if patient is taking beta blockers or calcium channel blockers. Signs, symptoms, and management can be similar to those for sepsis, severe sepsis, and septic shock.

Sepsis and Septic Shock

In sepsis, microorganisms invade the body. The result is SIRS that may lead to sepsis, ARDS, septic shock, MODS, and eventually death. Causes are gram-positive and gram-negative aerobes, anaerobes, fungi, and viruses. It is important to note that sepsis leading to septic shock and organ failure can occur along a continuum that may occur rapidly, causing death. Treatment and resuscitation should be started immediately upon diagnosis. Early recognition and intervention are crucial.

Pathophysiology

Sepsis is a condition in which organisms enter into the bloodstream and cause systemic activation of the host inflammation defense mechanism → release of cytokines and the activation of plasma protein cascade systems → septic shock → hypoperfusion of organs → multisystem organ failure. Massive vasodilation occurs in septic shock → ↓ peripheral vascular resistance → relative hypovolemia → ↓ venous return → ↓ stroke volume and cardiac output → insufficient organ perfusion → multisystem organ failure. A coagulation cascade is also activated causing platelets to adhere to the vascular endothelium → microthrombi → impede blood flow → microvascular hypoperfusion → inhibit O_2 to tissues, inhibit gas exchange → hypoxia and ischemia to major organs.

Patients with cancer in particular are at an increased risk of sepsis because of ↓ WBC, poor immune systems, and other contributing factors.

Clinical Presentation

- Temp >38°C (100.4°F) or <36°C (96.8°F)
- HR >90 bpm
- RR >20 bpm or Paco₂ <32 mm Hg
- WBC >12,000/mm³, <4,000/mm³, or >10% immature (band) forms
- Fever and chills
- Fatigue and malaise
- Warm and pink skin, progressing to cold, clammy, and mottled skin
- Significant edema or positive fluid balance (>20 mL/kg over 24 hr)
- Hypotension or normal BP: SBP <90 mm Hg or SBP decrease >40 mm Hg,
  MAP <70 mm Hg, leading to decrease in afterload and SVR
- Widening pulse pressure
- ↓ right atrial pressure (RAP) caused by decreased VR and preload and left
  ventricular stroke work index (LVSWI)
- Pao₂/Fio₂ ratio <300
- ↑ lactate levels and lactic acidosis
- Decreased urine output progressing to oliguria with ↑ serum creatinine levels
- Acute changes in mental status, such as anxiety, apprehension, delirium,
  disorientation, confusion, combativeness, agitation, lethargy, or coma
- Increased RR, SOB, crackles, hypoxemia progressing to pulmonary edema,
  acute lung injury, hypoxemia, and respiratory failure
- Nausea, vomiting, jaundice, ↑ GI motility, and ileus
- Changes in carbohydrate, fat, and glucose metabolism. Hyperglycemia
  >140 mg/dL in the absence of diabetes
- Signs of thrombocytopenia and coagulopathies (possibly progressing to DIC)
- Possible development of signs of septic shock

Diagnostic Tests

- CBC with differential (↑ or ↑ WBC). CBC may be normal but >10%
  immature (band) forms
- Platelet count and coagulation studies
- Basic metabolic panel, bilirubin (↑), serum lactate (↑), liver function tests
  (abnormal), amylase, and protein C (↑)
- Urinalysis and creatinine clearance
- 1,3-beta-D-glucan assay
- Anti-mannan antibody assays
- Plasma procalcitonin (PCT)
- Insulin resistance with elevated blood glucose
- ABGs (hypoxemia, lactic acidosis)
- ECG
- Urine, sputum, wound, and blood cultures
- Gram-Positive Blood Culture Nucleic Test (BC-GP)

234

- Coagulation studies including aPTT (↑), INR (↑), and D-dimer (↑)
- Imaging studies to confirm source of infection

Management

Management depends on the degree of sepsis and whether or not septic shock is present. Please refer to 2016 Society of Critical Care Medicine: www.survivingsepsis.org

Surviving Sepsis Campaign Care Bundles Based on the Surviving Sepsis Campaign Guidelines 2016

Within 3 hr of diagnosis of sepsis:

- Measure serum lactate level.
- Obtain at least two sets of blood cultures (both aerobic and anaerobic bottles) before antibiotic administration, one drawn percutaneously and one drawn through each vascular access device.
- Obtain BC-GP test if available.
- Administer broad-spectrum IV antibiotics within 1 hr of recognition of sepsis with or without shock. Reassess daily for effectiveness. Multidrug therapy often required. Administer antivirals as soon as indicated.
- If hypotension is present and/or serum lactate is ≥4 mmol/L, administer 30 mL/kg of crystalloid. Albumin recommended. Consider fluid challenge if hypovolemia suspected.

Within 6 hr of presentation with sepsis or septic shock:

- Insert arterial catheter for monitoring of BP.
- Administer vasopressors for hypotension not responding to fluid resuscitation to maintain MAP at ≥65 mm Hg. Norepinephrine (NE) is recommended as the first drug of choice. Dopamine tends to trigger arrhythmias.
- Add vasopressin 0.03 units/min to raise MAP or decrease NE dosage if needed as adjunct therapy to achieve MAP; not recommended as single initial vasopressor.
- Epinephrine may be added or substituted for NE if adjunct therapy is needed.
- Phenylephrine is recommended only if arrhythmias persist with other vasopressors or inotropes.
- Dopamine is not recommended for renal protection.
- Sodium bicarbonate therapy is not recommended for lactic acidemia with pH ≥7.15.
- Placement of arterial catheter (A-line) is highly recommended. Pulmonary artery catheter is not recommended.
- If arterial hypotension persists despite volume resuscitation or initial lactate ≥4 mmol/L (36 mg/dL), measure CVP and central venous oxygen saturation ($Scvo_2$).
- Remeasure lactate level if initial level was elevated.

MULTISYS

- Target guidelines include:
  - CVP 8–12 mm Hg
  - Scvo₂ >70%
  - MAP >65 mm Hg
  - Svo₂ saturation 65%
  - Urine output >0.5 mL/kg/hr
  - Lactate level within normal limits
  - Administer hydrocortisone IV only if hemodynamic instability persists.
  - Administer 200 mg/day by continuous flow. Taper drug when vasopressors are no longer required. Avoid ACTH stimulation test.
  - Transfuse patient with RBCs only when Hgb ≤7.0 g/dL. Target Hgb level is 7.0–9.0 g/dL in adults. Erythropoietin and fresh frozen plasma are not recommended.
  - Administer platelets if platelet count is <10,000/mm³.
  - Antithrombin administration is not recommended.
  - Selenium IV and IVIGs are not recommended.
  - Monitor serum procalcitonin levels; helps to define duration of antibiotic therapy.
  - Monitor for antibiotic-related diarrhea, especially caused by *Clostridium difficile.*
  - Start glucose control protocol if two consecutive blood glucose levels are >180 mg/dL. Target glucose level is <180 mg/dL.
  - Provide low-calorie oral or enteral feeding and advance as tolerated.
  - Consider IV glucose and enteral nutrition rather than solely TPN in the first 7 days after diagnosis.
  - Remove intravascular devices if deemed a source of infection.
  - Administer O₂ via nasal cannula, mask, or mechanical ventilation. Use minimum positive end-respiratory pressure to achieve tidal volume and end-inspiratory plateau pressure goals.
  - Follow protocols for mechanically ventilated patients; prevent ventilator-associated pneumonia (VAP). Refer to Basics and Respiratory Tabs.
  - Maintain a median inspiratory plateau pressure of ≤30 cm H₂O for mechanically ventilated patients.
  - Use PEEP as needed.
  - Avoid sodium bicarbonate for hypoperfusion-induced lactic acidemia pH ≥7.15.
  - Institute stress ulcer and DVT prophylaxis.
  - Sedate patient as necessary, but limit or avoid sedation when possible.
  - Consider train-of-four monitoring.
  - Consider CRRT and hemodialysis as needed.
  - Discuss goals of care and treatment with patient and family within 72 hr of ICU admission.
  - Use palliative care protocols where appropriate.
  - Refer to the reference section in the Tools Tab for complete guide.

Other Nursing Care

- Assess vital signs and monitor mean arterial pressure.
- Assess hemodynamic status. Refer to the previously noted target guidelines.
- Assess cardiac, respiratory, neurological, and GI status.
- Monitor ABGs and note ↓ pH, ↓ PaO_2, and ↑ $PaCO_2$. Monitor for ARDS. Refer to the Respiratory tab.
- Nurses should screen every patient for sepsis every shift using a sepsis screening tool. If a sepsis screen is positive, activate the rapid response team or rapid escalation of interventions using the 3-hr sepsis bundle.
- Assess and monitor anion gap and lactate if metabolic acidosis is present.
- Position patient to promote optimal O_2 exchange. Reposition every 2 hr.
- Keep head of bed (HOB) elevated 45°. Use prone position if possible.
- Institute VAP precautions if patient is on mechanical ventilation.
- Treat fever if present.
- Insert Foley catheter and monitor intake and output. Maintain urine output at ≥0.5 mL/kg/hr.
- Assess nutritional and fluid and electrolyte balance.
- Prevent nosocomial infections.
- Institute skin care protocols.

Shock

The four types of shock are:

- **Hypovolemic shock:** Resulting from decreased circulating or intravascular volume. Causes include hemorrhage, burns, acute pancreatitis, ascites, dehydration.
- **Cardiogenic shock:** Resulting from the inability of the heart to pump effectively. Causes include MI, cardiomyopathy, left-sided heart failure, blunt cardiac injury, acute mitral or aortic insufficiency.
- **Obstructive shock:** Resulting from a physical obstruction to blood circulation and inadequate blood oxygenation. Causes include pulmonary embolism, pneumothorax, aortic stenosis.
- **Distributive shock:** Resulting from maldistribution of circulating blood volume. Examples include:
  - Septic shock (caused by an infectious process)
  - Anaphylactic shock (a hypersensitivity reaction)
  - Neurogenic shock (from alterations in vascular smooth muscle tone)

Pathophysiology

The pathophysiology of shock is complex and not fully understood. It is characterized by hypoperfusion, hypercoagulability, and activation of the inflammatory response.

MULTISYS

- ↑ Blood volume displaced in the vasculature → ↓ cardiac output (CO) → ↑ HR and contractility with shunting of blood to the vital organs (brain).
- Renin-angiotensin response → angiotensin II (vasoconstriction) → release of aldosterone and antidiuretic hormone → Na+ and H₂O retention → ↑ preload.
- Stimulation of the anterior pituitary gland → secretion of adenocortico-tropic hormone → stimulation of adrenal cortex → release of glucocorti-coids → ↑ blood glucose.
- Stimulation of the adrenal medulla → release of epinephrine and norepinephrine → cell metabolism changes from aerobic to anaerobic → lactic acidosis.
- Cardiac hypoperfusion → ventricular failure.
- Cerebral hypoperfusion → failure of sympathetic nervous system, cardiac and respiratory depression, and thermoregulatory failure.
- Respiratory depression → ↑ pulmonary capillary membrane permeability → pulmonary vasoconstriction → acute respiratory failure and ARDS.
- Renal hypoperfusion → acute tubular necrosis → acute renal failure.
- GI hypoperfusion → failure of GI organs.
- MODS is failure of two or more body systems → death.

Clinical Presentation

- SBP <90 mm Hg. MAP <70 mm Hg and cardiac index <2.2 L/min/m², pulmonary wedge pressure >18 mm Hg, and systemic vascular resistance <1,400 dynes/sec/cm⁻⁵ in cardiogenic shock. Hypotension indicates >30% blood volume loss.
- ↑ HR, weak and thready pulse, narrowing of pulse pressure, dysrhythmias, absent peripheral pulses, dysrhythmias, chest pain.
- Delayed capillary refill and flat jugular veins. Distended neck veins are seen in cardiogenic shock.
- Altered mental status, confusion, altered level of consciousness (LOC) → lethargy and unconsciousness or unresponsiveness.
- Hypoxemia and respiratory alkalosis initially from RR and ↑ depth of respirations → respiratory failure → respiratory distress → respiratory and metabolic acidosis. Crackles or wheezing may also be present.
- Oliguria progressing to anuria, and ↓ urine osmolarity and specific gravity. Urine is dark and concentrated.
- ↑ BUN and creatinine.
- Pale and cool skin progressing to ashen, cold-clammy to cyanotic, mottled, and diaphoretic skin.

Hemodynamic Effects

Type of Shock	Preload	Afterload	Cardiac Output
Cardiogenic	↑	↑	↓
Hypovolemic	↓	↑	↓
Distributive	↓	↑↓	↓↑

Diagnostic Tests

Diagnosis and treatment of shock must be tailored to the cause.

- Serum chemistries, including electrolytes, BUN, and creatinine
- CBC and coagulation profile
- ABGs or pulse oximetry
- Cardiac output studies → ↓ CI, ↓ CO, ↓ preload, ↓ right atrial pressure (RAP), ↑ afterload, and ↑ systemic vascular resistance
- Cardiac markers may be useful: MB-CPK, troponin, BNP
- Serum lactate
- Urinalysis with specific gravity, osmolarity, and urine electrolytes. Urine C&S
- ECG
- Echocardiogram and cardiac angiography if cardiac origin
- CXR, CT, and ultrasound possibly helpful in identifying source of sepsis

Management

- Monitor vital signs and hemodynamics via arterial line and pulmonary artery catheter.
- Institute cardiac monitoring and treatment of dysrhythmias.
- Assess respiratory status and ABGs or pulse oximetry. Use of sodium bicarbonate has not been shown to be effective in treating lactic acidosis.
- Administer O_2 via cannula, mask, or mechanical ventilation. Assess for signs of hypoxia.
- Note skin color and temperature. Control fever.
- Assess neurological status and LOC.
- Administer IV fluids such as 0.9% NS and LR. Consider colloids and other crystalloids cautiously to prevent heart failure.
- Consider albumin and blood transfusions.
- Insert Foley catheter. Monitor intake and output.
- Assess fluid and electrolyte balance.

- Administer IV vasopressors as indicated by hemodynamic parameters.
- Maintain MAP ≥65 mm Hg and serum lactate >2 mmol/L (>18 mg/dL).
- Administer IV vasodilators and diuretics to ↓ preload or afterload.
- Administer sympathomimetics and digoxin to ↑ contractility.
- Administer antiarrhythmics if cardiac dysrhythmias are present. Consider cardioversion or a pacemaker if appropriate.
- Provide nutritional support, either enterally or parenterally.
- Institute intra-aortic balloon pump counterpulsation for cardiogenic shock or ventricular assist device. Consider percutaneous coronary intervention (PCI) or coronary artery bypass graft (CABG) to decrease myocardial workload and improve end-organ perfusion.
- Monitor serum lactic acid level. Administer sodium bicarbonate (not recommended in the treatment of shock-related lactic acidosis).
- Provide stress ulcer and DVT prophylaxis per institution policy and protocols.
- Provide analgesics for pain. Sedate as necessary.
- Provide emotional support to patient and family. Relieve anxiety.

Medications

Sympathomimetics are administered to improve contractility, ↑ SV, and ↑ CO:

- Dobutamine (Dobutrex)
- Dopamine (Intropin)
- Inamrinone (Amrinone)
- Milrinone (Primacor)
- Epinephrine (Adrenalin)
- Digoxin (Lanoxin)

Vasodilators are administered to ↑ preload and afterload and ↓ O_2 demand on the heart.

- Nitroglycerine (Tridil)
- Nitroprusside (Nipride)
- ACE inhibitors

Vasoconstrictors are administered to ↑ BP:

- Norepinephrine (Levophed)
- Phenylephrine (Neo-Synephrine)
- Vasopressin (Vasostrict)

Caution must be used in titrating medications to the patient's hemodynamic response.

Specific considerations for anaphylactic shock include:

- Administer an antihistamine or epinephrine.
- Administer corticosteroids or bronchodilators as indicated.
- Infuse crystalloid fluids over 1–3 min if patient is severely hypotensive or unresponsive to treatment.

Multiple Organ Dysfunction Syndrome (MODS)

MODS is defined as the physiological failure of two or more separate organ systems. The lungs are the most common organ to fail, followed by the kidneys and heart. With MODS, homeostasis cannot be maintained without specific interventions because of the body's inability to activate its own defense mechanisms sufficiently.

Those at high risk for developing MODS include patients with:

- Multiple trauma
- Massive infection or sepsis
- Hemorrhage or shock
- Surgical complications
- Acute pancreatitis
- Burns, extensive tissue damage, and/or necrotic tissue
- Aspiration
- Multiple blood transfusions
- Inadequate fluid resuscitation

Signs, symptoms, and management are similar to those for sepsis, severe sepsis, and septic shock. Initial organ failure includes the cardiovascular, pulmonary, and renal systems and can progress rapidly to the neurological, hematological, hepatic, metabolic, and GI systems.

- Monitor for decreasing SBP, MAP, O_2 saturation, urine output, platelets, bilirubin, alkaline phosphatase, aspartate aminotransferase, alanine aminotransferase, serum lactate, and a Glasgow Coma Scale <15 with changes in mental status.
- Monitor for increasing respiratory rate, coagulation times, and creatinine level.
- There is also an increased risk for DIC.
- The need for dialysis is an early warning sign of MODS.
- The Sequential Organ Failure Assessment score (SOFA score) can be calculated online at http://Clincalc.com/icumortality/sofa.aspx

Trauma

Pathophysiology

- **Blunt trauma:** Resulting from motor vehicle crashes (MVCs), falls, blows, explosions, contact sports, and blunt force injuries (e.g., from a baseball bat).
  - Estimating the amount of force a person sustains in an MVC = person's weight × miles per hour of speed.

- During an MVC, the body stops but the tissues and organs continue to move forward and then backward (acceleration-deceleration force).
- **Penetrating trauma:** Resulting from gunshot wounds, stabbings, and firearms or implement (missile, shrapnel) injuries.
  - There is direct damage to internal structures, with damage occurring along the path of penetration.
  - Penetrating trauma usually requires surgery.
- **Traumatic brain injury (TBI):** Resulting from a skull fracture, concussion, contusion, cerebral hematoma, and diffuse axonal injury.
- **Chest or thoracic injuries:** Resulting from either blunt trauma or a penetrating injury.
  - Common injuries include rib fractures, flail chest, ruptured diaphragm, aortic disruption, pulmonary contusion, tension or open pneumothorax, hemothorax, penetrating or blunt cardiac injuries, and cardiac tamponade.
- **Abdominal injuries:** Caused by blunt trauma or penetrating injury.
  - Common injuries include liver and spleen damage, renal trauma, bladder trauma, and pelvic fractures.
- **Musculoskeletal injuries:** Include spinal cord injury, fracture, dislocation, amputation, and tissue trauma.
  - Fat embolism may occur secondary to fractures of the long bones.

Diagnostic Tests

- CBC
- Serum chemistry panel, including electrolytes, glucose, BUN, and creatinine
- Liver function tests
- Serum amylase if pancreatic injury suspected or GI perforation is present
- Serum lactate level
- PT and PTT
- Urinalysis
- ABGs or pulse oximetry
- ECG
- Type and crossmatch for possible blood transfusion
- Drug and alcohol toxicology screens
- Pregnancy test for female patients of childbearing age
- X-rays specific to injury (e.g., chest, abdomen and pelvis, extremity)
- CT scan of the abdomen (ultrasound if indicated)
- Diagnostic peritoneal lavage if internal abdominal bleeding suspected
- Rectal or vaginal examination if indicated

Management

Management is highly dependent on the type of trauma.

- Maintain patent airway. Assess respiratory status for signs of trauma, tachypnea, accessory muscle use, tracheal shift, stridor, hyperresonance, dullness to percussion, rate depth, and symmetry.
- Monitor ABGs or pulse oximetry.
- Observe for respiratory distress and rising peak inspiratory pressure.
- Assess chest wall integrity for flail chest or pneumothorax.
- Administer O_2 via nasal cannula, mask, or mechanical ventilation. Use oropharyngeal or nasopharyngeal airway or endotracheal tube.
- Insert chest tube if pneumothorax is present.
- Assess for signs of bleeding. Control hemorrhage. Transfuse as needed. Consider autotransfusion of shed blood, autologous blood, unmatched type-specific blood, or type O (universal donor) blood.
- Consider pneumatic antishock garment to control hemorrhage.
- Replace each milliliter of blood loss with 3 mL of crystalloid (3:1 rule).
- Monitor vital signs frequently, and assess for signs of hypovolemic shock. Maintain BP within acceptable parameters.
- Provide continuous cardiac monitoring.
- Provide peripheral IV access or insert a central venous catheter for IV fluids. Use rapid infuser devices as needed.
- Assess neurological status for confusion and disorientation. Use Glasgow Coma Scale.
- Immobilize the spine and cervical area until assessment is made of spinal cord injury and head and neck injuries. If no injury, elevate HOB or turn patient to side to prevent aspiration.
- Prevent hypothermia through the use of blankets, warming blankets, or warming lights.
- Insert Foley catheter. Monitor intake and output. Assess fluid and electrolyte balance. Assess urine for bleeding.
- Assess abdomen. Note bowel sounds, guarding, bruising, tenderness, pain, rigidity, and rebound tenderness.
- Obtain focused abdominal sonography for trauma (FAST) followed by helical CT.
- Diagnostic peritoneal lavage (DPL) may be done if CT is not available or detects minimal abdominal fluid, if patient is unstable and needs immediate diagnosis of possible intra-abdominal hemorrhage, or if peritonitis is suspected. Most sensitive test for mesenteric and hollow viscus injuries. If >10 mL blood is aspirated, procedure stops and peritoneal cavity is lavaged with NS or LR; effluent sample is sent to the laboratory for analysis.
- Insert NG tube to prevent gastric distention, decrease risk of aspiration, and assess for GI bleeding.
- Provide nutritional support orally, enterally (gastric, duodenal, or jejunal route), or parenterally (TPN and lipids).
- Note skin color, pallor, bruising, distended neck veins, and edema.
- Inspect for soft tissue injury, deformities, wounds, ecchymosis, and tenderness. Palpate for crepitus and subcutaneous emphysema.

- All wounds should be thoroughly cleansed to the degree possible.
- Administer broad-spectrum antibiotics to prevent and treat infection.
- Observe for sepsis. Avoid nosocomial infections.
- Provide analgesics for pain. Sedate as necessary.
- Provide DVT and stress ulcer prophylaxis.
- Administer tetanus prophylaxis.
- Calculate and monitor a Trauma Score; https://www.easycalculation.com/medical/revised-trauma-score.php
- Calculate and monitor a Trauma Associated Severe Hemorrhage Score (TASH Score) for Massive Transfusion; https://www.mdapp.co/severe-hemorrhage-tash-score-calculator-183/

Complications

- Hypermetabolism; occurs 24 to 48 hr after traumatic injury
- Infection and sepsis; SIRS
- Acute respiratory failure or ARDS
- DVT; pulmonary or fat embolism
- Acute renal failure
- Compartment syndrome
- Dilutional coagulopathy
- MODS

Burns

Burns may be thermal, electrical, or chemical.

Type of Burn	Extent of Burn Injury	Description of Burn Injury
First-degree burn or superficial partial-thickness burn	• Epidermis destroyed	• Pinkish-red or red, dry • Usually not blistered • Blanching with pressure • Little or no edema • Tingling • Painful • Soothed by cooling
Second-degree burn: superficial partial-thickness	• Epidermis and upper layer of dermis destroyed	• Red or pink • Blistered, edema • Fluid exudate, "wet" • Hair follicles intact • Blanching with pressure • Sensitive to cold air • Very painful

Type of Burn	Extent of Burn Injury	Description of Burn Injury
Second-degree burn: deep partial-thickness	• Injury to deeper portions of dermis	
Third-degree or full-thickness burn	• Epidermis and dermis destroyed • May involve connective tissue, muscle, and bone • Underlying tissue may be destroyed	• Pale white, red, mottled • Broken skin with fat exposed • Edema or dry • No to slow blanching with pressure • Painless • Hair follicles and sweat glands destroyed
Fourth-degree or full-thickness burn	• Skin, fascia, muscle, and bone irreversibly destroyed	• Hard, dry, black, charred, cracked leather-like eschar • No pain or sensation • No blanching • Charred bones

A cold burn may occur when the skin is in contact with cold bodies (e.g., snow or cold air, as in cases of frostbite) or is exposed to dry ice or canned air. The treatment is the same for this type of burn.

Pathophysiology

Burns of <25% total body surface area (TBSA) → local response to injury.
Burns of >25% TBSA → local and systemic response to injury. Hypovolemia can develop if the burns involve >15%–20% of TBSA.
   There are three zones of thermal injury:

- Zone of coagulation (inner zone), where tissue necrosis is irreversible
- Zone of stasis (middle zone) surrounding the zone of coagulation
  - There is ↓ blood flow to the area and vascular damage.
  - Tissue damage may potentially be reversed with adequate care and treatment.
- Zone of hyperemia (outer zone) surrounding the zone of stasis
  - There is minimal injury to the area and evidence of early recovery.

Burn Stages
The two burn stages are the resuscitative phase and the acute phase.

Emergency or Resuscitative Phase

- The resuscitative phase begins at the time of injury and continues during the first 48–72 hr, until fluid and protein shifts are stabilized.
- Burn tissue injury occurs → loss of capillary integrity → ↑ permeability of capillary membrane → fluid shifts from the vascular to the interstitial spaces → ↓ cardiac output, ↓ BP, and ↑ HR and peripheral vasoconstriction → ↓ renal blood flow → ↓ renal function → acute renal failure.
- Fluid loss, ↓ renal blood flow, Na⁺ and water retention → ↓ urine output.
- Na⁺ and fluid pass through the burn areas → blisters, local edema, and fluid exudate → compartment syndrome.
- K⁺ is released from the tissue injury, and there is ↑ renal excretion of K⁺ → hyperkalemia.
- Lysis of RBCs occurs → hematuria, myoglobin in the urine, and anemia (↑ Hgb).
- Hemoconcentration → increase in Hct.
- Coagulation abnormalities occur → prolonged clotting and prothrombin times.
- Metabolic acidosis occurs.
- General tissue hypoperfusion results from ↓ circulating blood volume → burn shock → ↓BP and tachycardia.
- Hypothermia results from loss of skin barrier → thermoregulation problems.
- Associated inhalation injury may occur: carbon monoxide poisoning, injury above or below the glottis.

Intermediate or Acute Phase

- The acute phase of burn injury is characterized by the onset of diuresis. It generally begins approximately 48–72 hr after the burn injury and continues through near completion of wound closure. The last phase is the rehabilitation phase.
- Capillary membrane integrity returns → fluid shifts from interstitial to intravascular space → ↑ in blood volume → diuresis if good renal function exists.
- Fluid overload can occur.
- Hemodilution causes a ↓ in serum electrolytes and hematocrit.
- Na⁺ deficit may continue.
- K⁺ moves back into the cells → hypokalemia.
- Protein continues to be lost from the wound.

Diagnostic Tests

■ Calculation of TBSA injured according to the rule of nines:

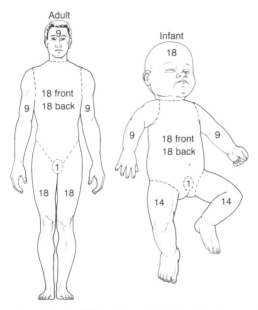

You can also calculate the TBSA of a burn with the Lund-Browder chart (most accurate method). Refer to http://frontlinefirstaid.ca/free-downloads/lund-and-browder-burn-chart-emr-bc-emalb.pdf

■ CBC
■ Serum chemistry panel, including electrolytes, glucose, BUN, and creatinine
■ Serum total protein and albumin
■ Liver function tests
■ Serum lactate level

- Carboxyhemoglobin level within 1 hr after injury
- CK and myoglobin levels possibly helpful
- PT and PTT
- Urinalysis (especially specific gravity, pH, glucose, acetone, protein, and myoglobin)
- ABGs or pulse oximetry and carboxyhemoglobin (COHgb)
- ECG
- Type and crossmatch for blood
- Drug and alcohol toxicology screens
- Pregnancy test for women of childbearing age
- X-rays specific to injury (e.g., chest, abdomen and pelvis, extremity)
- CT scan of abdomen (ultrasound if indicated)
- Bronchoscopy if inhalation injury is present

Management

Management of burns depends on the location and the extent of the burn injury.

- Maintain patent airway. Intubate or perform tracheostomy as needed.
- Administer 100% humidified O_2 by nasal cannula, mask, or mechanical ventilation/CPAP
- Assess respiratory status. Encourage the use of incentive spirometer, coughing and deep breathing, suctioning, or bronchodilators. Note respiratory distress.
- Monitor ABGs or pulse oximetry for hypoxemia and metabolic acidosis.
- Monitor COHgb levels.
- Monitor for and prevent pneumonia and other nosocomial infections.
- Immobilize the spine until assessment can be made of injury.
- Assess for inhalation injury.
- Irrigate chemical burns immediately.
- Control active bleeding if associated injuries.
- Assess TBSA burned and depth of burn injuries. Provide IV analgesics (opioids) for pain.
- Maintain good pain control. Consider ketamine and benzodiazepines before procedures.
- Initiate aggressive but cautious IV fluid resuscitation to replace fluid and electrolytes:
- Consensus Formula (Parkland Formula) recommendation is to give 4 mL/kg per percentage TBSA of lactated Ringer's solution in first 24 hr after burn injury.
- One half of the calculated total is given over the first 8 hr after burn injury, and the other half is given over the next 16 hr.

- Adjust fluids based on patient needs. Greatest volume fluid leak is in the first 24–36 hr after burn injury and peaks in 6–8 hr. Administer IV fluids cautiously if pulmonary or cerebral edema suspected.
  - Use of colloids controversial.
- Provide IV fluid boluses if ↓ BP, low urine output. Consider hemodynamic parameters and Hgb in view of patient's condition and comorbidities.
- Consider insertion of pulmonary artery catheter to monitor hemodynamics.
- Insert arterial line to monitor BP and obtain blood specimens. BP by cuff is inaccurate.
- Palpate peripheral pulses. Use Doppler if necessary.
- Provide continuous ECG monitoring.
- Insert NG tube if burn is >20% of the TBSA. Note GI bleeding.
- Assess GI status, noting bowel sounds, abdominal distention, and nausea. Administer antiemetics if nausea and vomiting present.
- Keep patient NPO initially. Assess nutritional status and provide feedings orally, enterally, or parenterally. Maintain aspiration precautions.
- Insert Foley catheter. Monitor intake and output with goal of 30–50 mL of urine/hr. Note hematuria. Burgundy-colored urine is composed of hemochromogen and myoglobin (hemoglobinuria and myoglobinuria).
- Consider bladder pressure monitoring if TBSA burn >30%.
- Weigh patient daily. Note height on admission to unit.
- Monitor electrolyte balance.
- Monitor serum glucose levels and treat per protocol.
- Assess neurological status for restlessness, confusion, difficulty concentrating, and changes in LOC.
- Assess warmth, capillary refill time, sensation, and movement of extremities.
- Keep HOB elevated 30°–45°. Elevate burned extremities.
- Monitor for infection and sepsis. Prevent nosocomial infection. Provide aseptic management of burn areas and invasive lines. Administer antibiotics as indicated.
- Burn patients may show signs and symptoms of SIRS that may be indicative of burn sepsis. Institute sepsis protocol if indicated.
- Provide DVT and stress ulcer prophylaxis.
- Administer tetanus vaccine prophylactically.
- Provide active and passive range-of-motion exercises.
- Treat anemia. Consider blood transfusions. Monitor coagulation factors.
- Provide warm environment through the use of clean sheets and blankets, or warm IV fluids.
- Monitor temperature, and prevent chills and shivering.
- Consider high-dose ascorbic acid in first 24 hr after burn.
- Provide psychosocial support to patient and family. Be alert for signs of depression. Provide antianxiety medications.
- In elderly patients, balance the risk of hypovolemia and fluid overload.

- In circumferential burns (burn completely surrounds body part), assess need for escharotomy, in which an incision is made through a full-thickness chest wound to decrease constriction, relieve pressure, and restore ventilation (chest) and/or improve blood flow and tissue perfusion.
- Refer to management of carbon monoxide toxicity in the Respiratory Tab.

Wound Care

- Cleanse wound as per protocol.
- Prepare patient for wound débridement (natural, mechanical, chemical, or surgical).
- Initiate topical antibacterial therapy:
  - Silver sulfadiazine (Silvadene) 1%
  - Silver nitrate aqueous solution ($AgNO_3$) 0.5%
  - Mafenide acetate (Sulfamylon) 5%–10%
  - Acticoat (silver-coated dressing)
  - Aquacel Ag (silver-coated dressing)
  - Silverlon (silver-coated dressing)
  - Mupirocin (antimicrobial)
  - Clotrimazole cream or nystatin (Mycostatin) if fungal infection is present
  - Diluted Dakin's solution
  - Petroleum-based ointments (bacitracin, gentamicin, neomycin)
- A vacuum-assisted closure (VAC) device may be used for wound healing along with a variety of dressings.

Patient/hospital-specific wound and dressing protocol

_____

_____

_____

_____

_____

_____

_____

_____

_____

_____

Wound Grafting and Wound Care Materials

Temporary impervious dressing materials: TransCyte. A variety of biological and synthetic skin grafts may be used for wound grafting:

- Homografts or allografts: Skin from another human, such as a cadaver
- Heterografts or xenografts: Skin from another animal, such as pigskin
- Autografts: Skin from oneself that is transferred from one part of the body to another
- Skin substitutes: Biobrane, Dermagraft, Integra, Apligraft, Matriderm, Orcel, Hyalomatrix, Renoskin, Kollagen, Matriderm, and AlloDerm

Complications

- Hypovolemia
- Decreased renal function, possibly leading to acute renal failure
- Infection and sepsis
- Paralytic ileus (decreased bowel sounds, distention, nausea, and vomiting)
- Curling's ulcer (stress ulcer or duodenal erosion)
- Metabolic acidosis
- Neurovascular compromise secondary to decreased blood flow to areas distal to the burn. It can result in tissue necrosis and possible amputation of extremity
- Hypothermia
- Acute respiratory failure and ARDS
- VAP
- Heart failure, pulmonary edema
- Sepsis
- Scarring
- Compromised immunity
- Changes in functional status, appearance, and body image, with associated depression
- Extremity compartment syndrome resulting from increased pressure in the fascial compartments of an extremity → compression and occlusion of blood vessels and nerves to the extremity. Symptoms include delayed capillary refill, tense skin, progressively diminishing or absent pulse to the extremity, intense pain, paresthesia, and paralysis of the extremity → ischemia and necrosis → loss of limb. Escharotomy is the treatment of choice. Eye orbital edema may require lateral canthotomy to reduce intraocular pressure.
- Abdominal compartment syndrome with symptoms including an increase in intra-abdominal pressure, tense abdomen, decreased urine output, hypercapnia, and difficulty with ventilation. This condition is treated by laparotomy, trunk escharotomies, and diuretics. Refer to GI Tab.

Commonly Used Critical Care Medications

This list is for reference use only and is not meant to replace any hospital policy or protocol. ALWAYS administer medications with caution in those patients with actual or suspected renal or liver impairment. The nurse is responsible for verifying all calculations before administering medications. This includes verifying dosages, concentrations, and titration policies with health care provider and facility pharmacy. Refer to hospital policies and procedures for most current information to ensure safe administration of drugs. Medication calculator that may be useful is found at http://www.globalrph.com/icudrip.htm

abciximab. Reopro: Antiplatelet agent, glycoprotein IIb/IIIa inhibitor. **Uses:** Prevention of cardiac ischemic complications in patients undergoing PCI; prevention of cardiac ischemic complications in patients with unstable angina/ NSTEMI unresponsive to conventional therapy when PCI is scheduled within 24 hr. **Dosages: Adult PCI: IV bolus** 0.25 mg/kg, administer 10–60 min before start of PCI by an infusion of 0.125 mcg/kg/min (max 10 mcg/min) for 12 hr; **Unstable angina/NSTEMI unresponsive to conventional medical therapy with planned PCI within 24 hr: IV bolus** 0.25 mg/kg followed by an 18–24 hr infusion of 10 mcg/min, concluding 1 hr after PCI.

adenosine. Adenocard: Antidysrhythmic. **Uses:** SVT, as a diagnostic aid to assess myocardial perfusion defects in CAD. **Usual dosages: IV bolus** 6 mg over 1–3 sec followed by rapid 20 mL NS flush. If conversion to NSR does not occur within 1–2 min, give 12 mg by rapid IV bolus; may repeat 12-mg dose again in 1–2 min. Administer via closest proximal port. A rapid 20-mL NS flush (as fast as possible) should be administered after each dose. Patient may be placed in mild reverse Trendelenburg position before giving drug and a rhythm strip recorded during administration.

alteplase. Activase: Thrombolytic enzyme. **Uses:** Lysis of obstructing thrombi associated with AMI, ischemic conditions requiring thrombolysis (i.e., PE, DVT), unclotting arteriovenous shunts, acute ischemic CVA). **Dosages:** >55 kg **IV** a total of 100 mg; 6–10 mg given **IV bolus** over 1–2 min, 60 mg given over first hr, 20 mg given second hr, 20 mg given over third hr. 1.25 mg/kg given over 3 hr for patients <65 kg.

amiodarone. Cordarone: Antidysrhythmic. **Uses:** Severe VT, SVT, atrial fibrillation, VF not controlled by first-line agents, cardiac arrest. **Dosages: PO** loading dose 800–1,600 mg/day for 1–3 wk; then 600–800 mg/day for 1 mo; maintenance 400 mg/day; **IV** loading dose (first rapid) 150 mg over the first 10 min, then slow 360 mg over the next 6 hr; maintenance 540 mg given over the remaining 18 hr, decrease rate of the slow infusion to 0.5 mg/min.

apixaban. Eliquis: Anticoagulant; Factor Xa inhibitor; direct oral anticoagulant. **Uses:** Deep vein thrombosis, nonvalvular atrial fibrillation, postoperative venous thromboprophylaxis, pulmonary embolism, conversion from one anticoagulant to another. **Dosages: PO** 10 mg twice daily for 7 days followed by 5 mg twice daily for DVT; **PO** 5 mg twice daily unless pt has any 2 of the following: Age ≥80 years, body weight ≥60 kg, or serum creatinine ≥1.5 mg/dL, then reduce dose to 2.5 mg twice daily for nonvalvular atrial fibrillation; **PO** 2.5 mg twice daily beginning 12–24 hours post-op for 35 days for hip replacement; **PO** 2.5 mg twice daily beginning 12–24 hours post-op for 12 days for knee replacement; **PO** 10 mg twice a day for 7 days followed by 5 mg twice daily for pulmonary embolism.

argatroban, **Argatroban:** Anticoagulant. Uses: Thrombosis, prophylaxis or treatment; PCI, anticoagulation prevention/treatment of thrombosis in heparin-induced thrombocytopenia. Dosages: ***Heparin-induced thrombocytopenia/thrombosis syndrome (HIT or HITTS):*** IV: 2 mcg/kg/min (1 mg/mL) give at 6 mL/hr for 50 kg, at 8 mL/hr for 70 kg, at 11 mL/hr for 90 kg, at 13 mL/hr for 110 kg, at 16 mL/hr for 130 kg. ***PCI in HIT:*** IV infusion 25 mcg/kg/min and a bolus of 350 mcg/kg given over 3–5 min, check ACT 5–10 min after bolus is completed; proceed if ACT >300 sec. ***Hepatic dose:*** **Continue infusion** 0.5 mcg/kg/min, adjust rate based on aPTT.

atenolol, **Tenormin:** Antianginal; beta blocker, beta-1 selective. Uses: Treatment of HTN, alone or in combination with other agents; management of angina pectoris; secondary prevention of MI. Dosages: **HTN:** **PO** 25–50 mg once daily, may increase to 100 mg/day: doses >100 mg are unlikely to produce any further benefit. **Angina pectoris:** **PO** 50 mg once daily; may increase to 100 mg/day. Some patients may require 200 mg/day. **Post MI:** **PO** 100 mg/day or 50 mg twice a day for 6–9 days.

atracurium, **Tracrium:** Neuromuscular blocker. Uses: Facilitation of tracheal intubation, skeletal muscle relaxation during mechanical ventilation, surgery, or general anesthesia. Dosages: **IV bolus** 0.3–0.5 mg/kg, then 0.8–0.10 mg/kg 20–45 min after first dose if needed for prolonged procedures.

atropine: Antidysrhythmic, anticholinergic, antimuscarinic. Parasympatholytic uses: Bradycardia, 40–50 bpm, bradydysrhythmia, reversal of anticholinesterase agents, insecticide poisoning, blocking cardiac vagal reflexes, decreasing secretions before surgery, antispasmodic with GU, biliary surgery, bronchodilator. Dosages: ***Bradycardia/bradydysrhythmias:*** IV bolus 0.5–1 mg given every 3–5 min, not to exceed 2 mg. ***Organophosphate poisoning:*** IM/IV 2 mg every hr until muscarinic symptoms disappear, may need 6 mg every hr. ***Presurgery*** SC/IM/IV 0.4–0.6 mg before anesthesia.

bivalirudin, **Angiomax:** Anticoagulant, thrombin inhibitor. Uses: Anticoagulant used in conjunction with aspirin for patients with unstable angina undergoing PTCA or PCI with provisional glycoprotein IIb/IIIa inhibitor; anticoagulant used in conjunction with aspirin for patient undergoing PCI with (or even at risk) for HIT/thrombosis syndrome (HITTS). Dosages: **IV bolus initially** 0.75 mg/kg immediately before procedure, followed by 1.75 mg/kg/hr for the duration of procedure and up to 4 hr post procedure if needed; may determine ACT 5 min after bolus dose: may administer additional bolus of 0.3 mg/kg if necessary. If continuous anticoagulation is needed after the initial 4-hr post-procedure infusion, the infusion may be continued at 0.2 mg/kg/hr for up

cisatracurium, **Nimbex**: Neuromuscular blocker agent, nondepolarizing. Uses: Adjunct to general anesthesia to facilitate endotracheal intubation and to relax skeletal muscles during surgery; to facilitate mechanical ventilation in ICU patients; does not relieve pain or produce sedation. Dosages: **Operating room administration: intubating dose IV** 0.15–0.2 mg/kg as components of propofol/nitrous oxide/oxygen induction-intubation technique. (Note: May produce generally good or excellent conditions for tracheal intubation in 1.5–2 min with clinically effective duration of action during propofol anesthesia of 55–61 min.) Initial dose after succinylcholine for intubation 0.1 mg/kg. **Maintenance dose IV** 0.03 mg/kg 40–60 min after initial dose, then at ~20-min intervals based on clinical criteria. **Continuous infusion: After initial bolus** a diluted solution can be given by continuous infusion for maintenance of neuromuscular blockade during extended surgery; adjust the rate of administration according to the patient's response as determined by peripheral nerve stimulation. An initial infusion rate of 3 mcg/kg/min may be required to rapidly counteract the spontaneous recovery of neuromuscular function; thereafter a rate of 1–2 mcg/kg/min should be adequate to maintain continuous neuromuscular block in the 89%–99% range in most patients. Spontaneous recovery from neuromuscular blockade following discontinuation of infusion of cisatracurium may be expected to proceed at a rate comparable to that following single bolus administration. **ICU administration:** Follow the principles for infusion in the operating room. At initial signs of recovery from bolus dose, begin the infusion at a dose of 3 mcg/kg/min and adjust rates accordingly. If patient is allowed to recover from neuromuscular blockade, readministration of a bolus dose may be necessary to re-establish blockade before reinstituting the infusion.

cosyntropin, **Cortrosyn**: Pituitary hormone. Uses: Testing adrenal cortical function. Dosage: **IM/IV** 0.25–1 mg between blood sampling.

dexmedetomidine, **Precedex**: Sedative, alpha-2-adrenoceptor agonist. Uses: Sedation in mechanically ventilated, intubated patients in the ICU. Dosages: **IV loading dose** of 1 mcg/kg over 10 min, then 0.2–0.7 mcg/kg/hr; do not use for more than 24 hr.

diltiazem, **Cardizem**: Calcium channel blocker. Uses: **IV** Atrial fibrillation, flutter, paroxysmal supraventricular tachycardia. Dosages: **IV bolus** 0.25 mg/kg over 2 min initially, then 0.35 mg/kg may be given after 15 min; if no response, may give **continuous infusion** 5–15 mg/hr for up to 24 hr.

dobutamine, **Dobutrex**: Adrenergic direct-acting beta-1-agonist, cardiac stimulant. Uses: Cardiac decompensation from organic heart disease or cardiac surgery. Dosages: **IV infusion** 2.5–10 mcg/kg/min; may increase to 40 mcg/kg/min if needed.

dopamine, **Intropin:** Adrenergic. Uses: Shock, increased perfusion, hypotension. Dosages: ***Shock:*** IV infusion 2–5 mcg/kg/min, not to exceed 50 mcg/kg/min, titrate to patient's response.

epinephrine: Bronchodilator nonselective adrenergic agonist, vasopressor. Uses: Acute asthmatic attacks, hemostasis, bronchospasm, anaphylaxis, allergic reactions, cardiac arrest, adjunction in anesthesia, shock. Dosages: ***Asthma:*** Inhaler 1–2 puffs of 1:100 or 2.25% racemic every 15 min. ***Bronchodilator:*** SC/IM 0.1–0.5 mg (1:1,000 sol) every 10–15 min–4 hr, max 1 mg/dose. ***Anaphylactic reaction/asthma:*** SC/IM 0.1–0.5 mg, repeat every 10–15 min, max 1 mg/dose; epinephrine suspension 0.5 mg **SC**, may repeat 0.5–1.5 mg every 6 hr. ***Cardiac arrest (ACLS):*** IV 1 mg every 3–5 min; **endotracheal** 2–2.5 mg; **intracardiac (IC)** 0.3–0.5 mg.

eptifibatide, **Integrilin:** Antiplatelet agent. Uses: Acute coronary syndrome including those undergoing PCI. Dosages: ***Acute coronary syndrome:*** IV **bolus** 180 mcg/kg as soon as diagnosed, then **IV Continuous** 2 mcg/kg/min until discharge or CABG up to 72 hr. ***PCI in patients without acute coronary syndrome:*** IV **bolus** 180 mcg/kg given immediately before PCI; then 2 mcg/kg/min for 18 hr and a second 180 mcg/kg bolus, 10 min after first bolus; continue infusion for up to 18–24 hr.

esmolol, **Brevibloc:** Beta-adrenergic blocker (antidysrhythmic II). Uses: SVT, noncompensatory sinus tachycardia, hypertensive crisis, intraoperative and postoperative tachycardia and HTN. Dosages: **IV loading dose** 500 mcg/kg/min over 1 min; maintenance 50 mcg/kg/min for 4 min; if no response in 5 min, give second loading dose; then increase infusion to 100 mcg/kg/min for 4 min; if no response, repeat loading dose, then increase maintenance infusion by 50 mcg/kg/min (max 200 mcg/kg/min), titrate to patient response.

etomidate, **Amidate:** General anesthetic. Use: Induction of general anesthesia. Dosages: **IV** 0.2–0.6 mg/kg over ½–1 min.

fenoldopam, **Corlopam:** Antihypertensive, vasodilator. Uses: Hypertensive crisis, malignant HTN. Dosages: **IV** 0.01–1.6 mcg/kg/min.

fentanyl, **Fentanyl:** Opioid analgesic. Uses: Preoperatively, postoperatively; adjunct to general anesthetic, adjunct to regional anesthesia; Fentanyl Oralet: Anesthesia as premedication, conscious sedation. Dosages: ***Anesthetic:*** IV 25–100 mcg (0.7–2 mcg/kg) every 2–3 min prn. ***Anesthesia supplement:*** IV 2–20 mcg/kg; **IV infusion** 0.025–0.25 mcg/kg/min. ***Induction and maintenance:*** IV **bolus** 5–40 mcg/kg. ***Preoperatively:*** IM 0.05–0.1 mg every 30–60 min before surgery. ***Postoperatively:*** IM 0.05–0.1 mg every 1–2 hr prn.

haloperidol, **Haldol:** Antipsychotic agent, typical. Uses: labeled indications: Management of schizophrenia; control of tics and vocal utterances of Tourette's disorder in children and adults; severe behavioral problems in children. Unlabeled uses: Treatment of non-schizophrenia psychosis; may be used for the emergency sedation of severely agitated or delirious patients; treatment of ICU delirium; adjunctive treatment of ethanol dependence; postoperative nausea and vomiting (alternative therapy);

psychosis/agitation related to Alzheimer's dementia. Dosages: **Psychosis:**
PO 0.5–5 mg 2–3 times/day; usual max 30 mg/day. **IM** (as lactate): 2–5 mg
every 4–8 hr as needed. **IM** (as decanoate): Initial 10–20 times the daily oral
dose administered at 4-wk intervals. Maintenance dose: 10–15 times initial
oral dose; used to stabilize psychiatric symptoms. **Delirium in the ICU, treat-**
ment (unlabeled use, unlabeled route): **IV** initial dose 0.5–10 mg depending
on degree of agitation; if inadequate response, may repeat bolus dose
(with sequential doubling of initial bolus dose every 15–30 min until calm
is achieved, then administer 25% of the last bolus dose every 6 hr; monitor
ECG and QTc interval. After the patient is controlled, haloperidol therapy
should be tapered over several days. **Delirium in the ICU (patients at high**
risk of delirium), prevention (unlabeled use, unlabeled route): **IV** 0.5 mg followed by a continuous infusion of 0.1 mg/hr for 12 hr **or** of 0.5 mg every 8 hr.
Rapid tranquilization of severely agitated patient (unlabeled use: administer
every 30–60 min): **PO** 5–10 mg. **IM** (as lactate) 5 mg. Average total dose (oral
or IM) for tranquilization: 10–20 mg. Average total dose **Postoperative nausea and vomiting**
(unlabeled use): **IM, IV** 0.5–2 mg.

heparin. **Heparin.** Anticoagulant. Uses: labeled indications: Prophylaxis and
treatment of thromboembolic disorders; as an anticoagulant for extracorporeal and dialysis procedures. Unlabeled uses: STEMI as an adjunct
to thrombolysis; unstable angina/NSTEMI; anticoagulant used during PCI.
Dosages: **Acute coronary syndromes—IV infusion** (weight-based dosing per
institutional nomogram recommended): STEMI, **as adjunct to fibrinolysis:**
Initial bolus of 60 units/kg (max: 4,000 units) then 12 units/kg/hr as continuous infusion. Check aPTT every 4–6 hr: adjust to target of 1.5–2 times the
upper limit of control (50–60 sec). Duration of heparin therapy depends on
concurrent therapy and the specific patient risks for systemic or venous
thromboembolism. **Unstable angina: IV bolus** initially 60 units/kg, followed
by an initial infusion of 12 units/kg/hr. Check aPTT every 6 hr: adjust to
target rate of 1.5–2 times the upper limit of control (50–70 sec). Continue
for 48 hr in low-risk patients managed with a conservative strategy. **PCI:** No
prior anticoagulation therapy. **If no GPIIb/IIIa inhibitor use planned: IV bolus**
70–100 units, kg **or if planning GPIIb/IIIa inhibitor use:** IV bolus of 50–70 units/kg.
Prior anticoagulation therapy. **If no GPIIb/IIIa inhibitor use:** additional
heparin as needed **or** if planning GPIIb/IIIa inhibitor use: additional heparin
as needed. **Thromboprophylaxis (low-dose heparin): SC** 5,000 units every
8–12 hr. **Treatment of venous thromboembolism:** Start warfarin on the first
or second treatment day and continue heparin until INR is ≥2 for at least
24 hr (usually 5–7 days).

ibutilide. **Corvert.** Antiarrhythmic agent, class III. Uses: Acute termination of
atrial fibrillation or flutter of recent onset. Dosages: **Atrial fibrillation/**
flutter: IV <60 kg: 0.01 mg/kg over 10 min. >60 kg: 1 mg over 10 min. **Note:**
Discontinue infusion if arrhythmia terminates, if sustained or nonsustained
VT occurs, or if marked prolongation of QT/QTc occurs. If the arrhythmia

does not terminate within 10 min after the end of the initial infusion, a second infusion of equal strength may be infused over a 10-min period.

isoproterenol, **Isuprel:** Beta-adrenergic agonist. Uses: Bronchospasm, asthma, heart block, ventricular dysrhythmias, shock. Dosages: *Asthma, bronchospasms:* SL 10–20 mg every 6–8 hr, max 60 mg/day; INH 1 puff, may repeat in 2–5 min, maintenance 1–2 puffs 4–6 times/day; IV 10–20 mcg during anesthesia. *Shock:* IV infusion 0.5–5 mcg/min. 1 mg/500 mL D5W, titrate to BP, CVP, hourly urine output.

labetalol, **Normodyne:** Antihypertensive, antianginal. Uses: Mild to moderate HTN; treatment of severe HTN. Dosages: *HTN:* PO 100 mg twice a day; may be given with a diuretic; may increase to 200 mg twice a day after 2 days; may continue to increase every 1–3 days; max 2,400 mg/day in divided doses. *Hypertensive crisis:* IV infusion 200 mg/160 mL D5W, infuse at 2 mL/min; stop infusion at desired response, repeat every 6–8 hr as needed; IV bolus 20 mg over 2 min, may repeat 40–80 mg every 10 min, not to exceed 300 mg.

lidocaine: Antidysrhythmic (class Ib). Uses: Ventricular tachycardia, ventricular dysrhythmias during cardiac surgery, MI, digitalis toxicity, cardiac catheterization. Dosages: IV bolus 50–100 mg (1 mg/kg) over 2–3 min, repeat every 3–5 min, not to exceed 300 mg in 1 hr; begin IV infusion. IV infusion 20–50 mcg/kg/min; IM 200–300 mg (4.3 mg/kg) in deltoid muscle, may repeat in 1–1½ hr if needed.

lorazepam, **Ativan:** Benzodiazepine. Uses: labeled indications: PO management of anxiety disorders or short-term (<4 mo) relief of symptoms of anxiety, anxiety associated with depressive symptoms, or insomnia related to anxiety or transient stress. IV status epilepticus, amnesia, sedation. Unlabeled indications: Ethanol detoxification; psychogenic catatonia; partial complex seizures; agitation; antiemetic for chemotherapy; rapid tranquilization of the agitated patient. Dosages: **Antiemetic:** PO, IV 0.5–2 mg every 4–6 hr as needed. **Anxiety, sedation, and procedural amnesia:** PO 1–10 mg/day in 2–3 divided doses; usual dose 2–6 mg/day in divided doses or 1–2 mg 1 hr before procedure. IM 0.05 mg/kg administered 2 hr before surgery (max dose 4 mg). IV 0.044 mg/kg 15–20 min before surgery (usual dose 2 mg; max dose 4 mg). **Insomnia:** PO 2–4 mg at bedtime. **Status epilepticus:** IV 4 mg/dose slowly (max rate 2 mg; max dose 4 mg). **Rapid tranquilization of agitated patient** (unlabeled use): PO, IM 1–2 mg administered every 30–60 min. **Agitation in the ICU patient** (unlabeled use): IV loading dose: 0.02–0.04 mg/kg (max single dose 2 mg); maintenance 0.02 mg–0.06 mg/kg every 2–6 hr as needed **or** 0.01–0.1 mg/kg/hr. **Alcohol withdrawal syndrome** (unlabeled use): PO 2 mg every 6 hr for 4 doses, then 1 mg every 6 hr for 8 additional dosages. **Alcohol withdrawal delirium** (unlabeled use): IV 1–4 mg every 5–15 min until calm, then every hr as needed to maintain light somnolence. IM 1–4 mg every 30–60 min until calm, then every hr as needed to maintain light somnolence.

magnesium sulfate: Anticonvulsant, miscellaneous, electrolyte supplement, parenteral; magnesium salt. Uses: Treatment and prevention of hypomagnesemia; prevention and treatment of seizures in severe pre-eclampsia or eclampsia, torsade de pointes; treatment of cardiac arrhythmias (VT/VF) caused by hypomagnesemia; soaking aid. **Dosages:** Dose represented as magnesium sulfate unless stated otherwise. **Hypomagnesemia—Mild magnesium deficiency: IM** 1 g every 6 hr for 4 doses, or as indicated by serum magnesium concentrations. **Severe magnesium deficiency: IM** up to 250 mg/kg within a 4-hr period. Severe non–life-threatening deficiency: **IV** 1–2 g/hr for 3–6 hr then 0.5 g/hr as needed to correct deficiency. **Symptomatic magnesium deficiency: IV** 1–2 g over 50–60 min: maintenance infusion may be required to correct deficiency (0.5–1 g/hr). **Polymorphic VT (including torsades de pointes): IV push** 1–2 g; **Seizures** 1–2 g over 10 min. **Eclampsia: IV** 4–5 g infusion: followed by a 1–2 g/hr continuous infusion or may follow with **IM** 4–5 g in each buttock every 4 hr. **Pre-eclampsia (severe): IV infusion** 4–5 g; followed by a 1–2 g/hr continuous infusion or may follow with **IM** doses of 4–5 g in each buttock every 4 hr; max dose 40 g/24 hr. **Torsades de pointes or VF/pulseless VT associated with torsades de pointes: IV, IO:** 1–2 g over 15 min or faster with cardiac arrest. **Parenteral nutrition supplementation: IV** 8–24 mEq elemental magnesium/day.

metoprolol, **Lopressor:** Antianginal agent; beta-1 selective. **Uses:** **Labeled indications:** Treatment of angina pectoris, HTN, or hemodynamically stable AMI. **Unlabeled indications:** Treatment of ventricular arrhythmias, atrial ectopy, migraine prophylaxis, essential tremor, prevention of reinfarction and initial: multifocal atrial t...cardia; symptomatic treatment of hypertrophic obstructive cardiomyopathy, management of thyrotoxicosis. **Dosages: PO** *immediate release:* initial: 50 mg twice/day, max dose 400 mg/day; increase dose at weekly intervals to desired effect. *Extended release:* initial: 100 mg/day (max 400 mg/day). **Atrial fibrillation/flutter (ventricular rate control), SVT: IV** 2.5–5 mg every 2–5 min (max total dose: 15 mg over a 10–15 min period). Maintenance **PO** *immediate release* 25–100 mg twice daily. **Heart failure: PO** *extended release:* initial: 25 mg once daily; may double dosage every 2 wk as tolerated. **HTN PO** *immediate release:* initial: 50 mg twice daily, increase dose at weekly intervals to desired effect, max dose 450 mg/daily. *Extended release:* initial: 25–100 mg once daily, increase doses at weekly intervals to desired effect. Max dose 400 mg/daily. **HTN/ventricular rate control: IV** initial dose 1.25–5 mg every 6–12 hr: titrate initial dose to response. **AMI: IV** 5 mg every 2 min for 3 doses in early treatment of MI, thereafter give 50 mg **PO** every 6 hr beginning 15 min after last IV dose and continue for 48 hr, then a maintenance dose of 100 mg twice daily. **Thyrotoxicosis: PO** *immediate release* 25–50 mg every 6 hr.

midazolam, **Versed:** Sedative, hypnotic, antianxiety. **Uses:** Preoperative sedation, general anesthesia induction, sedation for diagnostic endoscopic procedures, intubation. Dosages: **Preoperative sedation:** **IM** 0.07–0.08 mg/kg 1/2–1 hr before general anesthesia. **Induction of general anesthesia:** **IV** (unpremedicated patients) 0.3–0.35 mg/kg over 30 sec, wait 2 min, follow with 25% of initial dose if needed; (premedicated patients) 0.15–0.35 mg/kg over 20–30 sec, allow 2 min for effect. **Continuous infusion for intubation (critical care):** **IV** 0.01–0.05 mg/kg over several min; repeat at 10–15 min intervals, until adequate sedation; then 0.02–0.10 mg/kg/hr by continuous infusion; adjust as needed.

milrinone, **Primacor:** Inotropic/vasodilator agent with phosphodiesterase activity. Uses: Short-term management of advanced CHF that has not responded to other medication; can be used with digitalis. Dosages: **IV bolus** 50 mcg/kg given over 10 min; start infusion of 0.375–0.75 mcg/kg/min; reduce dose in renal impairment.

naloxone, **Narcan:** opioid-agonist, antidote. Uses: Respiratory depression induced by opioids, pentazocine, propoxyphene; refractory circulatory shock, asphyxia neonatorum, coma, hypotension. Dosages: **Opioid-induced respiratory depression:** **IV/SC/IM** 0.4–2 mg; repeat every 2–3 min if needed. **Postoperative opioid-induced respiratory depression:** **IV** 0.1–0.2 mg every 2–3 min prn. **Opioid overdose:** **IV/SC/IM** 0.4 mg (10 mcg/kg) (not opioid dependent), may repeat every 2–3 min (opioid dependent).

nesiritide, **Natrecor:** Vasodilator. Uses: Acutely decompensated CHF. Dosages: **IV bolus** 2 mcg/kg, then **IV infusion** 0.01 mcg/kg/min nitroglycerine: Coronary vasodilator, antianginal. Uses: Chronic stable angina pectoris prophylaxis of angina pain, CHF associated with AMI, controlled hypotension in surgical procedures. Dosages: SL, transdermal, topical doses available. IV infusion uses listed only **IV** 5 mcg/min, then increase by 5 mcg/min every 3–5 min; if no response after 20 mcg/min, increase by 10–20 mcg/min until desired response

nicardipine, **Cardene:** Antianginal agent; calcium channel blocker, dihydropyridine. Uses: Chronic stable angina (immediate release product only); management of HTN (immediate and sustained release products); IV only for short-term use only when oral treatment not feasible. Dosing: **Angina: Immediate release, PO** 20 mg 3 times/day; usual range 60–120 mg/day; increase dose at 3-day intervals. **HTN: PO** immediate release initial dose 20 mg 3 times a day; usual dose 20–40 mg 3 times a day (allow 3 days between dose increases). **Sustained release:** Initial 30 mg twice a day. **Acute HTN:** **IV** initial dose 5 mg/hr increased by 2.5 mg/hr every 5 min (for rapid titration) to every 15 min (for gradual titration) up to max of 15 mg/hr; rapidly titrated patients, consider reduction to 3 mg/hr after response is achieved.

nitroglycerin: Antianginal agent, vasodilator. Uses: Labeled indications: Treatment or prevention of angina pectoris. Unlabeled indications: Short-term management of pulmonary HTN, esophageal spastic disorders, uterine relaxation. Dosages: **Angina/coronary artery disease: PO** 2.5–6.5 mg 3–4 times/daily. **IV** 5 mcg/min, increase by 5 mcg/min every 3–5 min to

20 mcg/min. If no response at 20 mcg/min, may increase by 10-20 mcg/min every 3-5 min. Topical ointment 1/2 inch-2 inches every 6 hr; patch, transdermal 0.2-0.4 mg/hr initially and titrate to doses of 0.4-0.8 mg/hr (tolerance is minimized by using patch 12-14 hr/day and off 10-12 hr/day SL 0.3-0.6 mg every 5 min for max of 3 doses in 15 min; may also use prophylactically 5-10 min before activities that may provoke an attack. Translingual 1-2 sprays onto or under tongue every 3-5 min for max of 3 doses in 15 min, may also be used prophylactically 5-10 min before activities that may provoke an angina attack. Esophageal spastic disorders: SL 0.3-0.5 mg. Uterine relaxation: IV bolus 100-200 mcg; may repeat dose every 2 min as necessary.

nitroprusside. Nitropress: Antihypertensive, vasodilator. Uses: Hypertensive crisis, to decrease bleeding by lowering hypotension during surgery, acute heart failure. Dosages: IV infusion dissolve 50 mg in 2-3 mL of D5W, then dilute in 250-1,000 mL of D5W; infuse at 0.5-8 mcg/min.

norepinephrine. Levophed: Adrenergic. Uses: Acute hypotension, shock. Dosages: IV infusion 8-12 mcg/min titrated to BP.

pancuronium. Pavulon: Neuromuscular blockade. Uses: Facilitation of endotracheal intubation, skeletal muscle relaxation during mechanical intubation, surgery or general anesthesia. Dosages: IV 0.04-0.1 mg/kg, then 0.01 mg/kg every ¼-1 hr.

phenylephrine. Neo-Synephrine: adrenergic, direct acting. Uses: Hypotension, paroxysmal SVT, shock, maintain BP for spinal anesthesia. Dosages: Hypotension: SC/IM 2-5 mg, may repeat every 10-15 min if needed, do not exceed initial dose; IV 50-100 mcg, may repeat every 10-15 min if needed, do not exceed initial dose. SVT: IV bolus 0.5-1 mg given rapidly, not to exceed prior dose by >0.1 mg, total dose ≤1 mg. Shock: IV infusion 10 mg/500 mL D5W given 100-180 mcg/min, then maintenance of 40-60 mcg/min.

procainamide. Pronestyl: Antidysrhythmic. Uses: Life-threatening ventricular dysrhythmias. Dosages: Atrial fibrillation/PAT: PO 1-1.25 g; may give another 750 mg if needed; if no response, 500 mg-1 g every 2 hr until desired response; maintenance 50 mg/kg in divided doses every 6 hr. Ventricular tachycardia: PO 1 g; maintenance 50 mg/kg/day given in 3-hr intervals; sustained release 500 mg-1.25 g every 6 hr. Other dysrhythmias: IV bolus 100 mg every 5 min, given 25-50 mg/min, not to exceed 500 mg; or 17 mg/kg total, then IV infusion 2-6 mg/min.

propofol. Diprivan: General anesthetic. Uses: Induction or maintenance of anesthesia as part of balanced anesthetic technique; sedation in mechanically ventilated patients. Dosages: Induction IV 2-2.5 mg/kg, approximately 40 mg every 10 sec until induction onset. Maintenance IV 0.1-0.2 mg/kg/min (6-12 mg/kg/hr); ICU sedation: IV 5 mcg/kg/min over 5 min; may give 5-10 mcg/kg/min over 5-10 min until desired response.

rivaroxaban, Xarelto: Anticoagulant, Factor Xa inhibitor, direct oral anticoagulant. Uses: Deep vein thrombosis, pulmonary embolism treatment and reduction in risk of recurrent DVT/PE after at least 6 mo of initial anticoagulation, post-op DVT prophylaxis, nonvalvular atrial fibrillation, conversion from one anticoagulant to another. Dosage: **PO** 15 mg twice a day with food for 21 days followed by 20 mg once a day with food for DVT/PE treatment, 10 mg once daily for recurrent DVT/PE after anticoagulation, 10 mg daily 6–10 hr post-op for minimum 10–14 days for knee replacement and 10 mg daily for 35 days for hip replacement, 20 mg daily with evening meal for nonvalvular atrial fibrillation, for conversion, initiate as soon as INR <3.0.

rocuronium, **Zemuron:** Neuromuscular blocker (nondepolarizing). Uses: Facilitation of endotracheal intubation, skeletal muscle relaxation during mechanical ventilation, surgery or general anesthesia. Dosages: ***Intubation:*** **IV** 0.6 mg/kg.

streptokinase, **Streptase:** Thrombolytic enzyme. Uses: DVT, PE, arterial thrombosis, arteriovenous cannula occlusion, lysis of coronary artery thrombi after MI, acute evolving transmural MI. Dosages: ***Lysis of coronary artery thrombi:*** **IC** 20,000 units, then 2,000 international units/min over 1 hr as **IV infusion.** ***Arteriovenous cannula occlusion:*** **IV** infusion 250,000 international units/2 mL solution into occluded limb of cannula run over ½ hr; clamp for 2 hr, aspirate contents; flush with NaCl solution and reconnect. ***Thrombosis/embolism/DVT/pulmonary embolism:*** **IV** infusion 250,000 international units over 1/2 hr, then 100,000 international units/hr for 72 hr for deep vein thrombosis; 100,000 international units/hr over 24–72 hr for pulmonary embolism; 100,000 international units/hr over 24–72 hr for arterial thrombosis or embolism. ***Acute evolving transmural MI:*** **IV** infusion 1,500,000 international units diluted to a volume of 45 mL; give within 1 hr; intracoronary **infusion** 20,000 international units by **bolus,** then 2,000 international units/min for 1 hr, total dose 140,000 international units.

succinylcholine, **Anectine:** Neuromuscular blocker (depolarizing–ultrashort). Uses: Facilitation of endotracheal intubation, skeletal muscle relaxation during orthopedic manipulations. Dosages: **IV** 0.6 mg/kg, then 2.5 mg/min as needed; **IM** 2.5 mg/kg, not to exceed 150 mg.

tenecteplase, **TNKase:** Thrombolytic enzyme. Use: AMI. Dosages: *Adult <60 kg:* **IV** bolus 30 mg, give over 5 sec. *Adult <70 kg:* **IV** bolus 35 mg, give over 5 sec. *Adult ≥70–<80 kg:* **IV** bolus 40 mg, give over 5 sec. *Adult ≥80–<90 kg:* **IV** bolus 45 mg, over 5 sec. *Adult ≥90 kg:* **IV** bolus 50 mg, give over 5 sec.

tirofiban, **Aggrastat:** Antiplatelet. Use: Acute coronary syndrome in combination with heparin. Dosages: **IV** 0.4 mcg/kg/min × 30 min, then 0.1 mcg/kg/min for 12–24 hr after angioplasty or atherectomy.

tubocurarine, **Tubarine:** Neuromuscular blocker. Uses: Facilitation of endotracheal intubation, skeletal muscle relaxation during mechanical ventilation, surgery or general anesthesia. Dosages: **IV** bolus 0.4–0.5 mg/kg, then 0.8–0.10 mg/kg 20–45 min after first dose if needed for long procedures.

urokinase, **Abbokinase:** Thrombolytic enzyme. Uses: Venous thrombosis, PE, arterial thrombosis, arterial embolism, arteriovenous cannula occlusion, lysis of coronary artery thrombi after MI. Dosages: *Lysis of pulmonary emboli:* **IV 4,400 international units/kg/hr for 12–24 hr,** not to exceed 200 mL; then **IV heparin, then anticoagulants.** *Coronary artery thrombosis:* **Instill 6,000 international units/min into occluded artery for 1–2 hr after giving IV bolus of heparin 2,500–10,000 units. May also give as IV infusion 2 million–3 million units over 45–90 min.** *Venous catheter occlusion:* **Instill 5,000 international units into line, wait 5 min, then aspirate; repeat aspiration attempts every 5 min for 1/2 hr; if occlusion has not been removed, cap line and wait 1/2–1 hr, then aspirate; may need second dose if still occluded.** **Pitressin:** Pituitary hormone, vasoconstrictor. Uses: Diabetes insipidus (non-nephrogenic/nonpsychogenic), abdominal distention postoperatively, bleeding esophageal varices, sepsis. Dosages: *Diabetes insipidus:* **IM/SC 5–10 units 2–4 times a day as needed.** *Abdominal distention:* **IM 5 units, then 2–3 days for long-term therapy.** *Sepsis IV infusion 0.03 units/hr, may titrate to 0.04 units/hr for BP.*

verapamil. Calan: Antianginal agent, antiarrhythmic agent (class IV), calcium channel blocker, calcium channel blocker-nondihydropyridine. Uses: Labeled indications: Treatment of HTN, angina pectoris, SVT. Unlabeled indications: Hypertrophic cardiomyopathy, bipolar disorder. Dosages: *Angina PO immediate release initial 80–120 mg 3 times/day. Extended release* initial 180 mg once daily at bedtime; if inadequate response, may increase dose at weekly intervals to 240 mg once daily, then 360 mg once daily, then 480 mg once daily. *Chronic atrial fibrillation (rate-control), PSVT prophylaxis:* **PO** *immediate release* 240–480 mg/day in 3–4 divided doses. HTN: **PO** *immediate release* 80 mg 3 times/day. *Sustained release* 120–140 mg/day in 1–2 divided doses. *Extended release* usual dose range 120–360 mg once daily. SVT: **IV 2.5–5 mg over 2 min;** second dose of 5–10 mg may be given 15–30 min after the initial dose.

Symbols and Abbreviations

↑ ....increase(d)
↑↑ ....greatly increased
↓ ....decrease(d)
↓↓ ....greatly decreased
→ ....leads to, causes
≤ ....less than or equal to
≥ ....greater than or equal to
/ ....per, or, divided by
% ....percent
(–) ....negative
(+) ....positive
° .... degree(s)
mc ....micro
A-a.............................alveolar-arterial
AAA....... abdominal aortic aneurysm
AAD.................... antibiotic-associated diarrhea
Ab... antibody
ABG......................... arterial blood gas
ACE ....angiotensin-converting enzyme
ACE-I........... angiotensin-converting enzyme inhibitor
AChr.................acetylcholine receptor
ACS .... acute coronary syndrome or abdominal compartment syndrome
ACT..............activated coagulation time
ACTH.................... adrenocorticotropic hormone
ACV .... assist controlled ventilation
ADH.................... antidiuretic hormone
AgNO₃............. silver nitrate aqueous solution
AICD...............automatic implantable cardioverter defibrillator device
AIS.................... acute ischemic stroke
AKI............................acute kidney injury
ALI......................... acute lung injury
A-line..................................arterial line
AMI.........acute myocardial infarction

ANA....................antinuclear antibody
APP.....................abdominal perfusion pressure
aPTT.........................activated partial thromboplastin time
ARB.. ....angiotensin receptor blocker
ARDS..........adult respiratory distress syndrome
ASA...aspirin
AV.................... atrial-ventricular
AVM..........arteriovenous malformation
BCP.................birth control pills
BE....................................base excess
BiPAP ....bilevel positive airway pressure
BIVAD..........right and left ventricular assist device
BM.................... bowel movement
BMI....................... body mass index
BMP.....................basic metabolic panel
BNP .... B-type natriuretic peptide
BP ....blood pressure
BPD .... billopancreatic diversion/ bypass
bpm ....breaths or beats per minute
BPS..................Behavioral Pain Scale
BSA ....body surface area
BSI.....................bispectral index monitoring
BUN/CR............. blood urea nitrogen/ creatinine
C ....Celsius or cervical spine
Ca²⁺..calcium
CABG ....coronary artery bypass graft
CAD............................coronary artery disease
CAM-ICU........ Confusion Assessment Method for the Intensive Care Unit

CAP	community acquired pneumonia	CPR	cardio-pulmonary resuscitation
CAPP	coronary artery perfusion pressure	CRP	c-reactive protein
CAUTI	catheter-associated urinary tract infection	CRRT	continuous renal replacement therapy
CASS	continuous aspiration of subglottic secretions	CRT	cardiac resynchronization therapy
CAVH	continuous arteriovenous hemofiltration	C&S	culture and sensitivity
CAVHDF	continuous arteriovenous hemodifiltration	CSF	cerebrospinal fluid
CBC	complete blood count	CT(A)	computed tomography (angiograph)
C&DB	cough and deep breathe	CVA	cerebrovascular accident
CE	carotid endarterectomy	CVP	central venous pressure
CHO	carbohydrates	CVVH	continuous venovenous hemofiltration
CI	cardiac index		
CK	creatine kinase	CVVHDF	continuous venovenous hemodiafiltration
CK-MB	creatine kinase myocardial band	CXR	chest x-ray
CLABSI	central catheter-associated bloodstream infection	DBP	diastolic blood pressure
		DDS	Delirium Detection Scale
CLRT	continuous lateral rotation therapy	DI	diabetes insipidus
cm	centimeter	DIC	disseminated intravascular coagulation
CMP	complete metabolic panel	DKA	diabetic ketoacidosis
CMV	continuous mandatory ventilation	dL	deciliter
		DNI	do not intubate
CN	cranial nerve	DNR	do not resuscitate
CNS	central nervous system	Do₂	oxygen delivery
CO	cardiac output, carbon monoxide	DOE	dyspnea on exertion
		DPL	diagnostic peritoneal lavage
CO₂	carbon dioxide	DSA	digital subtraction angiography
COHgb	carboxyhemoglobin		
COP	colloid osmotic pressure	DVT	deep vein thrombosis
COPD	chronic obstructive pulmonary disease	D/W	dextrose in water
		D5W	5% dextrose in water
CPAP	continuous positive airway pressure	EBCT	electron beam computed tomography
CPIS	clinical pulmonary infection score	ECG	electrocardiogram
		EC-IC	extra-intracranial bypass
CPOT	Critical Care Pain Observation Tool	ECMO	extracorporeal membrane oxygenator
CPP	cerebral perfusion pressure	ED	emergency department
		EEG	electroencephalogram

e.g. ....for example
EIA....................enzyme immunoassay
EjFx or EF ....ejection fraction
EMG ....electromyelogram
EP ....electrophysiology
ESCRF ....end-stage chronic renal failure
ESKD ....end-stage kidney disease
ESR............erythrocyte sedimentation rate
$ETCO_2$............end-tidal carbon dioxide
ETOH.....................................alcohol
ETT ....endotracheal tube
F...Fahrenheit
FAST..........Focused abdominal sonography for trauma
FIO_2 ....fraction of inspired oxygen
FDP................fibrin degradation product
FENa....... fractional excretion sodium
FEUrea ....fractional excretion urea
FFP.....................fresh frozen plasma
FRC........ functional residual capacity
g ....gram
GBS............ Guillain-Barr syndrome
GFR .... glomerular filtration rate
GI..gastrointestinal
GRV(s)...... gastric residual volume(s)
GU... genitourinary
GYN..............gynecology, gynecological
H^+ .... hydrogen ion
HAIs ....hospital-acquired (nosocomial) infections
hCG ....human chorionic gonadotropin
HCO_3^- ....bicarbonate ion
Hct..hematocrit
HF ....heart failure
HFJV......................high-frequency jet ventilation
HFOV.......... high-frequency oscillatory ventilation
HFPPV ....high-frequency positive pressure ventilation
Hgb.....................................hemoglobin

HIT.........................heparin-induced thrombocytopenia
HLA ....human leukocyte antigen
H_2O ....water
HOB.......................................head of bed
HR..heart rate
hr...hour(s)
HRT .... hormone replacement therapy
HSS ..... hyperosmolar hyperglycemic state
HTN...............................hypertension
Hx..history
IABP ....intra-aortic balloon pump
IAH ......intra-abdominal hypertension
IAP .... intra-abdominal pressure
IC .... intracardiac (route of administration)
ICDSC...........Intensive Care Delirium Severity Checklist
ICP .... intracranial pressure
ICU ....intensive care unit
I.D. ....internal diameter
IM...............................intramuscular(ly)
IMA............................ischemia modified albumin
INR ....international normalized ratio
IO.......................................intraosseous
IRV...............inverse ratio ventilation
IV.......................................intravenous(ly)
IVIG .....intravenous immune globulin
IVP.....................intervenous pyelogram
J...joules
JVD............jugular venous distention
K^+ ....potassium
kg ....kilogram
KUB.................kidney-ureters-bladder
L............... liter or lumbar spine
LAP.......................left atrial pressure
LMWH........low molecular weight heparin
LOC ....level of consciousness
LPGD ....low-profile gastrostomy device

LR	lactated Ringer's solution
LV	left ventricle
LVAD	left ventricle assist device
LVEDP	left ventricular end-diastolic pressure
LVF	left ventricular failure
LVSWI	left ventricular stroke work index
m	meter
max	maximum
MAP	mean arterial pressure
mcg	microgram
mEq	milliequivalent
mg	milligram
MG	myasthenia gravis
MI	myocardial infarction
MIDCAB	minimally invasive direct coronary artery bypass graft
min	minute
mL	milliliter
mm	millimeter
mm Hg	millimeters of mercury
mmol	millimole
MODS	multiple organ dysfunction syndrome
MRA	magnetic resonance angiography
MRI	magnetic resonance imaging
MS	musculoskeletal
msec	millisecond
MUGA	MRI with gadolinium
MV	minute ventilation
MVC	motor vehicle crash
Na^+	sodium
NaCl	sodium chloride
$NaHCO_3$	sodium bicarbonate
NDT	nasoduodenal tube
NE	norepinephrine
NGT	nasogastric tube
NIMC	noninvasive mechanical ventilation

NJT	nasojejunal tube
NMBA	neuromuscular blocking agent
nmol	nanomole
NPO	nothing by mouth
NS	normal saline
NSAIDs	nonsteroidal anti-inflammatory drugs
NSR	normal sinus rhythm
NSTEMI	non-ST-segment elevation myocardial infarction
NTG	nitroglycerin
NVPS	Nonverbal Adult Pain Assessment Scale
O_2	oxygen
OOB	out of bed
OSA	obstructive sleep apnea
PAC	premature atrial contraction
$Paco_2$	partial pressure of carbon dioxide in arterial blood
PAD	pulmonary artery diastolic pressure
PAH	pulmonary arterial hypertension
Pao_2	partial pressure of oxygen in arterial blood
PAO_2	partial pressure of alveolar oxygen
PAP	pulmonary artery pressure
PAP_m	mean pulmonary artery pressure
PAS	pulmonary artery systolic pressure
PASG	pneumatic antishock garment
PAT	paroxysmal atrial tachycardia
$PbTO_2$	partial pressure of brain tissue oxygen
PCI	percutaneous coronary intervention

PCO_2	partial pressure of carbon dioxide
PCV	pressure controlled ventilation
PCWP	pulmonary capillary wedge pressure
PE	pulmonary embolism
PEA	pulseless electrical activity
PEEP	positive end-expiratory pressure
PEG	percutaneous endoscopic gastrostomy
PEJ	percutaneous endoscopic jejunostomy
PET	positron emission tomography
PFT	pulmonary function tests
P/F ratio	PAO_2/FIO_2
pH	potential of hydrogen
PO	by mouth, orally
Po_2	partial pressure of oxygen
PPI	proton pump inhibitor
PPV	positive pressure ventilation
PQRST	palliative/provoking, quality, radiation, severity, timing
PRBC	packed red blood cells
prn	as needed
PSV/PS	pressure support ventilation
PTCA	percutaneous transluminal coronary angioplasty
PT/PTT	prothrombin time/partial thromboplastin time
PVC	premature ventricular contraction
PVR	pulmonary vascular resistance
PVRI	pulmonary vascular resistance index
RA	right atrium
RAP	right atrial pressure
RASS	Richmond Agitation Sedation Scale
RBBB	right bundle branch block
RBCs	red blood cells
REM	rapid eye movement
RF	rheumatoid factor
RR	respiratory rate
RRT	renal replacement therapy
RSI	rapid sequence induction
RSWI	right ventricular stroke work index
rtPA	recombinant tissue plasminogen activator
RV	right ventricle
RVAD	right ventricular assist device
RVF	right ventricular failure
RVSW	right ventricular stroke work
SAH	subarachnoid hemorrhage
Sao_2	oxygen saturation
SAS	Sedation Agitation Scale
SBO	small bowel obstruction
SBP	systolic blood pressure
SC	subcutaneous(ly)
SCI	spinal cord injury
SCUF	slow continuous ultrafiltration
Scvo_2	central venous oxygen saturation
SE	status epilepticus
sec(s)	second(s)
SGOT	serum glutamic oxaloacetic transaminase
SGPT	serum glutamic pyruvic transaminase
SI	stroke index
SIADH	syndrome of inappropriate antidiuretic hormone
SIMV	synchronous intermittent mandatory ventilation
SIRS	systemic inflammatory response syndrome
Sjvo_2	cerebral or jugular venous oxygen saturation
SL	sublingual
SOB	shortness of breath
sol	solution

SPECT	single-photon emission computed tomography
SpO₂	saturation of peripheral oxygen via pulse oximetry
SRA	serotonin release assay
STAT	immediately
STEMI	ST-segment elevation myocardial infarction
SV	stroke volume
SVCS	superior vena cava syndrome
SvO₂	systemic venous oxygen saturation
SVR	systemic vascular resistance
SVT	supraventricular tachycardia
T	thoracic spine
VAPS	volume assured pressure support
TAVR	transcatheter aortic valve replacement
TBI	traumatic brain injury
TBSA	total body surface area
TCD	transcranial Doppler
TEE	transesophageal echocardiogram

Temp	temperature
TIA	transient ischemic attack
TnI	troponin I
TOF	train of four
TPN	total parenteral nutrition
TSH	thyroid-stimulating hormone
UA	urinalysis
UGI	upper gastrointestinal
UTI	urinary tract infection
VAC	vacuum-assisted closure
VAD	ventricular assist device
VAP	ventilator-associated pneumonia
VAS	Visual Analog Scale
VF	ventricular fibrillation
VO₂	oxygen consumption
vol	volume
V/Q	ventilation:perfusion
VR	venous return
VS	vital signs
VT	ventricular tachycardia
V–V	venous-venous
WBC	white blood cell count

Troubleshooting ECG Problems

- Place leads in the correct position. Incorrect placement can give false readings.
- Avoid placing leads over bony areas.
- In patients with large breasts, place the electrodes under the breast. Accurate tracings are obtained through the least amount of fat tissue.
- Shave hair at the electrode site if it interferes with contact between the electrode and skin.
- Prevent ECG alarm fatigue and false alarms by:
  - Providing proper skin preparation for ECG electrodes such as washing the electrode areas with soap and water, wiping with rough gauze or washcloth
  - Changing the electrodes daily
  - Customizing the alarm parameters to the patient

Patient ECG Record

Patient name:_____

Sex   F   M

Heart rate: _____ bpm

- Normal (60–100 bpm)   Y   N
- Bradycardia (<60 bpm)   Y   N
- Tachycardia (>100 bpm)   Y   N

Rhythm

- Regular   Y   N
- Irregular   Y   N
- P waves   Y   N

P waves (form)

- Normal (upright and uniform)   Y   N
- Inverted   Y   N

P wave associated with QRS   Y   N
PR interval normal (0.12–0.20 sec) Y   N
P waves and QRS complexes associated with one another Y   N

QRS interval

- Normal (0.6–0.10 sec)   Y   N
- Wide (>0.10 sec)   Y   N

Are the QRS complexes grouped or not grouped?
Are there any dropped beats?
Is there a compensatory or noncompensatory pause?

QT interval: _____

Interpretation: _____

_____

Patient's medications that may cause ECG changes: _____

Patient's blood chemistries or electrolytes that may cause ECG changes: ____

Contributing past medical or surgical history or co-morbidities: _____

Frequently Used Phone Numbers

Overhead Code:	99/Blue:
Rapid Response Team:	
Fire:	
Security:	Emergency ext:
Other emergency:	
Admitting:	
Behavioral Health:	
Blood Bank:	
Burn Unit:	
Cardiothoracic or Cardiovascular ICU:	
Coronary Care Unit (CCU):	
Medical ICU (MICU):	
Neuro ICU:	
Respiratory ICU (RICU):	
Surgical ICU (SICU):	
Trauma ICU:	
Other ICUs:	
Chaplain-Pastor-Pastoral Care:	
Computer Help (IS, IT):	
CT (Computed Tomography):	
Dietary—Dietician:	
ECG—12-Lead:	
Housekeeping:	
Infection Control:	
Interventional Radiology:	
Laboratory:	
Maintenance—Engineering:	
Med-Surg Units/Telemetry:	
MRI (Magnetic Resonance Imaging):	
Nutrition—Food Services:	

Continued

OT (Occupational Therapy):	
PACU (Recovery):	
Pediatrics:	
Pharmacy (Rx):	
Poison Control:	USA – 1-800-222-1222
PT (Physical Therapy):	
Respiratory (RT):	
Social Services:	
Speech Language Pathology (SLP):	
Supervisor—Manager:	
Surgery—Inpatient (OR):	
Surgery—Day/Outpatient:	
X-ray:	

Community Resources

Abuse/Assault—Physical/Sexual	
• Children	
• Women	
• Rape/sexual	
• Men	
• Elderly	
Abuse—Substance	
• Alcohol	
• Drug	
Communicable Disease Programs	
• AIDS	
• Hepatitis	

Continued

Mental Health	
• Suicide	
Medical/Hospitals	
• State program	
• Dept. of Health	
• Free clinics	
Other	

Basic English-to-Spanish Translation

English Phrase	Pronunciation	Spanish Phrase
Introductions—Greetings		
Hello	**oh**-lah	Hola
Good morning	**bweh**-nohs **dee**-ahs	Buenos d as
Good afternoon	**bweh**-nohs **tahr**-dehs	Buenos tardes
Good evening	**bweh**-nahs **noh**-chehs	Buenas noches
My name is	*meh **yah**-moh*	Me llamo
I am a nurse	soy lah oon en-fehr-**meh**-ra	Soy la enfermera
What is your name?	**koh**-moh seh **yah**-mah oo-**sted**?	¿ Cómo se llama usted?
How are you?	**koh**-moh eh-**stah** oo-**stehd**?	¿Como esta usted?
Very well	*mwee b' yehn*	Muy bien
Thank you	**grah**-s'yahs	Gracias
Yes, no	**see**, noh	Sí, no
Please	pohr fah-**vohr**	Por favor
You're welcome	deh **nah**-dah	De nada

Continued

English Phrase	Pronunciation	Spanish Phrase
Assessment—Areas of the Body		
Head	kah-**beh**-sah	Cabeza
Eye	**oh**-hoh	Ojo
Ear	oh-**ee**-doh	O do
Nose	nah-**reez**	Nariz
Throat	gahr-**gahn**-tah	Garganta
Neck	**kweh**-yoh	Cuello
Chest, heart	**peh**-choh, kah-rah-**sohn**	Pecho, coraz n
Back	eh-**spahl**-dah	Espalda
Abdomen	ahb-**doh**-mehn	Abdomen
Stomach	eh-**stoh**-mah-goh	Est mago
Rectum	**rehk**-toh	Recto
Penis	**peh**-neh	Pene
Vagina	vah-**hee**-nah	Vagina
Arm, hand	**brah**-soh, **mah**-noh	Brazo, mano
Leg, foot	p'**yehr**-nah, p'**yeh**	Pierna, pie
Assessment—History		
Do you have...	T'**yeh**-neh oo-**stehd**...	¿Tiene usted...
Difficulty breathing?	di-fi-kul-**thad** par-rehspee-**rahr**	¿Dificultad para respirar?
Chest pain?	doh-**lorh** en el **peh**-chow	¿Dolor en el pecho?
Abdominal pain?	doh-**lorh** ab-doh-mee-**nahl**	¿Dolor abdominal?
Diabetes?	dee-ah-**beh**-tehs	¿Diabetes?
Are you...	ehs-**tah**	¿Esta...
Dizzy?	mar-eh-**a**-dho(dha)	¿Mareado(a)?
Nauseated?	kahn **now**-say-as	¿Con nauseas?
Pregnant?	¿ehm-bah-rah-**sah**-dah?	¿Embarazada?
Allergic to any medications?	¿ehs ah-**lehr**-hee-koh ah ahl-**goo**-nah meh-dee-**see**-nah?	¿Es alergico a alguna medicina?

Continued

Assessment—Pain

English Phrase	Pronunciation	Spanish Phrase
Do you have pain?	**T'yeh**-neh oo-**stehd** doh-**lorh**?	¿Tiene usted dolor?
Where does it hurt?	dohn-deh leh **dweh**-leh?	¿Donde le duele?
Is the pain...	es oon doh-lor...	¿Es un dolor...
Dull?	**Leh**-veh	¿Leve?
Aching?	kans-**tan**-teh	¿constante?
Crushing?	ab-**plahs**-tan-teh?	¿Aplastante?
Sharp?	ah-**goo**-doh?	¿Agudo?
Stabbing?	ah-**poo**-nya-lawn-teh	¿Apu alante?
Burning?	Ahr-**d'yen**-the?	¿Ardiente?
Does it hurt when I press here?	Leh dweh-**leh** kwahn-doh ah-pree-eh-toh ah-**kee**?	¿Le duele cuando le aprieto aqui?
Does it hurt to breathe deeply?	S'yen-teh oo-**sted** doh-lor **kwahn**-doh reh-spee-rah pro-foon-dah-**men**-teh?	¿Siente usted dolor cuando respira profundamente?
Does it move to another area?	Lh doh-**lor** zeh moo-eh-veh a oh-tra **ah**-ri-ah	¿El dolor se mueve a otra area?
Is the pain better now?	S'yen **ley** al-goo-nah me-**horr**-ee-ah	¿Siente alguna mejor a?

Online Translation Programs

- Google Translate: https://translate.google.com
- BabelFish: https://babelfish.com
- Oxford Dictionary Translation: https://en.oxforddictionaries/com/definition/translation

Communication With a Nonverbal Patient

Pain	1	2	3	4	5	6	7	8	9	10

Yes	No	Thank You

Cold	Hot	Sick

Thirsty	Hungry

Please Bring:	Empty:
■ Blanket	■ Bed Pan
■ Eyeglasses	■ Urinal
■ Dentures	■ Trash
■ Hearing Aids	Raise – Lower:
	■ Head
	■ Legs

Oral Care	Bath	Shower

TV	Lights	On	Off

TOOLS

Common Laboratory Values

The following lab values are a representation of normal values and their equivalents. Always refer to your facility's laboratory reference guide to determine whether a value is WNL, as normal value parameters vary slightly for each lab.

Serum Chemistries and Electrolytes

Value	Normal Range	Equivalent
Albumin	3.5–5.0 g/dL	35–55 g/L
Alkaline Phosphatase (ALP)	38–126 U/L	0.5–1.5 µKat/L
Ammonia	15–45 mcg/dL	11–35 SI units
Amylase	60–160 Somogyi unit/dL	30–170 SI units
Bilirubin, Direct	0.1–0.3 mg/dL	1.7–5.1 SI units
Bilirubin, Total	0.1–1.2 mg/dL	1.7–20.5 SI units
BUN	10–25 mg/dL	2.5–8.0 mmol/L
Calcium	9–11 mg/dL	2.3–2.8 units
Chloride	95–105 mEq/l	95–105 SI units
Creatinine	0.5–1.5 mg/dL	45–132.3 SI units
Glucose	60–100 mg/dL	3.3–5.8 mmol/L
Lactate	4–16 mg/dL	0.5 2.0 mmol/L
Magnesium	1.5–2.5 mEq/L	1.8–3.0 mg/dL
Osmolarity	280–300 mOsm/kg	280–300 mmol/kg
Phosphorus	1.7–2.6 mg/dL	0.78–1.52 SI units
Potassium	3.5–5.3 mEq/L	3.5–5.3 SI units
SGOT (AST)/SGPT (ALT)	10–35 units/L	4–36 SI units
Sodium	135–145 mEq/L	135–145 SI units
Total Protein	6.0–8.0 g/dL	60–78 g/L
Uric Acid	2.8–8.0 mg/dL	0.15–0.47 mmol/L

Hematology

Value	Normal Range
Basophils	0.4%–1.0% = 40–100 mm^3
Eosinophils	1%–3% = 100–300 mm^3
Erythrocyte Sedimentation Rate	0–20
Hemoglobin (varies by gender)	M: 13.5–16.5 g/dL F: 12.0–15.0 g/dL
Hematocrit (varies by gender)	M: 41%–50% F: 36%–44%
Lymphocytes	25%–35% = 1,700–3,500 mm^3
Monocytes	4%–6% = 200–600 mm^3
Neutrophils (total)	50%–70% = 2,500–7,000 mm^3
Platelets	150,000–400,000 µL
RBC (varies by gender)	M: 4.5–5.5 × 10^5/mL F: 4.0–4.9 × 10^5/mL
WBC	4,500–10,000 mm^3

Therapeutic Drug Levels

Value	Toxic Level	Equivalent
Carbamazepine (Tegretol)	15 µg/mL	64 µmol/L
Digoxin (Lanoxin)	>2.5 ng/mL	>3.2 nmol/L
Dilantin (Phenytoin)	10–20 mcg/mL	39.6–79.3 SI units
Phenobarbital (Solfoton)	>40 µg/mL	>172 µmol/L
Tobramycin	>10 µg/mL	>21 µmol/L
Valproic Acid (Depakene)	>200 µg/mL	>1,400 µmol/L
Vancomycin	>80 µg/mL	>54 µmol/L

Urine

Value	Normal Range
Osmolarity	50–1,200 mOsm/kg/H_2O
pH	4.5–8
Specific Gravity	1.010–1.030

Cerebral Spinal Fluid

Value	Normal Range	Equivalent
Protein	15–60 mg/dL	150–600 mg/L
Glucose	40–80 mg/dL	2.5–4.4 mmol/L
Leukocytes (Total)	<5/mm3	
Color	Clear, colorless	
Cell Count	0–5 cells/µL	0–0.5×106 cells/L
Specific Gravity	1.006–1.008	

Arterial Blood Gas Normal Values – Refer to Basics Tab
Coagulation Values – Refer to Hem/Onc Tab

Web Resources for Evidence-Based Practices in Critical Care

Agency for Healthcare Research and Quality .... www.ahrq.gov
American Association of Critical-Care Nurses .... www.aacn.org
American Association of Neuroscience Nurses .... www.aann.org/
American College of Cardiology .... www.cardiosource.org/acc
American Heart Association .... www.heart.org
American Society for Parenteral and
    Enteral Nutrition .... www.nutritioncare.org/
American Stroke Association .... www.strokeassociation.org
American Thoracic Society ....www.thoracic.org
Centers for Disease Control and Prevention .... www.cdc.gov
Critical Care Nutrition .... www.criticalcarenutrition.com/

Illustration Credits

Pages 89 and 101: From Jones, J: ECG Notes, ed. 2. F.A. Davis, Philadelphia, 2010.

Pages 95, 96, and 102: From Hopkins, T: MedSurg Notes, ed. 3. F.A. Davis, Philadelphia, 2011.

Pages 98–100 and 103–107: From Armstrong Medical Industries, Inc. Lincolnshire, IL.

Pages 145 and 247: From Myers E: RNotes, 5th ed. F.A. Davis, Philadelphia, 2018.

Index